to yesteryear's tiresome and stodgy health and wellness tomes—and most important, it's one hell of a good time."

—Rochelle Bilow, editor at *Bon Appétit* and author of *The Call of the Farm*

"A vast compendium of knowledge that informs, debunks, amuses you—and disabuses you of the notion that kale is awesome."

—Brian Sack, TV host and author of *The B.S. of A.* and *In the Event of My Untimely Demise*

"Interrupting the endless swirl of information telling us we're doing it wrong or we're doing it right, Jeff Wilser's book is a calming, hilarious, and information-packed reminder that everything should be taken with a grain of salt (and maybe a shot of whiskey, too)."

—Jen Doll, author of *Save the Date: The Occasional Mortifications of a Serial Wedding Guest*

THE
GOOD
NEWS

ABOUT WHAT'S BAD FOR YOU

THE
GOOD
NEWS

ABOUT WHAT'S BAD FOR YOU

JEFF WILSER

FLATIRON
BOOKS
NEW YORK

www.flatironbooks.com

Interior illustrations © David Curtis Studio
Interior design by Michelle McMillian
Cover design by Karen Horton
Cover illustrations © Shutterstock

The Library of Congress Cataloging-in-Publication Data is available
upon request.

ISBN 978-1-250-06380-9 (hardcover)
ISBN 978-1-250-06381-6 (e-book)

Our books may be purchased in bulk for promotional, educational, or business use.
Please contact your local bookseller or the Macmillan Corporate and
Premium Sales Department at (800) 221-7945, extension 5442,
or by e-mail at MacmillanSpecialMarkets@macmillan.com.

First Edition: December 2015

10   9   8   7   6   5   4   3   2   1

To everyone who has ever felt guilty about
eating red meat,
drinking bourbon,
or not buying organic

Contents

AUTHOR'S NOTE

This is not a how-to guide to health. Use it for informational purposes only. Consult with your doctor before making any changes. Read labels and warnings carefully, avoid extremes, and always listen to your body. (In other words, please don't start a Twinkie diet.)

Introduction

Eat more bacon. Drink more whiskey. Take more naps.

This advice isn't mine; this is the advice from science. In study after study, trial after trial, a new crop of research says that much of what's "bad for us" is one of three things: 1) not as bad as we thought; 2) not bad at all; 3) actually good for us.*

Exhibit A: fat. If you're a human who was born between 1940 and 2010, you've been told that Eating Fat=Bad. *Fat raises cholesterol. Fat causes heart attacks. Fat makes us fat.* The government officials, who wore lab coats and pointed to charts and graphs, sure seemed pretty confident. So we tried to obey. Despite shrieks of protest from our taste buds, we held our noses and swapped butter for

---

*Kind of. Sort of. The world of health is tricky, it's nuanced, and it's filled with asterisks. We'll get to the many disclaimers in a bit.

margarine, cooked with vegetable oil, and scooped up groceries labeled "fat-free."

Only one little problem: as we cut down on fat we loaded up on sugar. The new evidence convicts sugar, not fat, as the criminal who plumped the nation. Diets high in fat can beat their low-fat counterparts. Eggs are making a glorious comeback. New research—especially the work of Gary Taubes and Nina Teicholz, who we'll hear from—suggests that the original premise of the low-fat craze, *saturated fat causes heart disease*, was flawed from its inception.

Judging by headlines like "Butter Is Back" in the *New York Times* and "Let Them Eat Fat" in the *Wall Street Journal,* this once-renegade idea has gone mainstream. "It's time to end the low-fat myth. For decades, a low-fat diet was touted as a way to lose weight and prevent or control heart disease and other chronic conditions, and food companies re-engineered products to be reduced-fat or fat-free, often compensating for differences in flavor and texture by increasing amounts of salt, sugar, or refined grains. However, as a nation, following a low-fat diet hasn't helped us control weight or become healthier." These aren't the words of some fringe doctor; they're from Harvard's School of Public Health.

Exhibit B: gluten. It's true that for people with celiac disease (roughly 1 percent of the population), it's crucial to avoid gluten. For the other 99 percent of us, racing into the arms of gluten-free substitutes, cooked with unholy additives, can spur us to eat food that's even junkier. This fad, like most fads, can backfire. (But just to be safe, this book is made from paper that's 100 percent gluten-free.)

Exhibit C: salt. We're told to curb our intake, even though the risk of heart attack—the Big Threat—is highest for those with *low* levels of sodium.

Exhibit D: junk food. Many new studies suggest that . . . okay, well, there aren't any studies that exonerate junk food. It's called junk for a reason. But maybe, in moderation, cookies aren't as bad as we think? In the name of science, for thirty days I ate nothing but these four food groups:

- Junk food
- Black coffee
- Protein shakes
- Whiskey

I ate no fruit, no vegetables, no cheese, no legumes, no whole grains. No real food at all. Oreos for breakfast, Snickers for lunch, Cracker Jack for dinner. Thirty days of this. I felt fine. I lost 11 pounds.

Why does all this matter?

If we continue to follow outdated advice, we'll continue to make poor choices. Science evolves. Humans, as a species, are still in a very, very early chapter in the book of medicine. Yesterday's truths are tomorrow's regrets. Doctors once spiked cough syrup with heroin, cured patients with "a good bleeding," kept a straight face while they performed lobotomies, and told our grandparents that it's fine to puff cigarettes. As recently as the 1970s, homosexuality was "treated" with shock therapy. We learn from mistakes.

This very second, across the globe, teams of scientists race to find new data, conduct new trials, and launch new studies. Rats scurry in labs. Doctors check pulses. Volunteers pee in cups. Each study hopes to improve our understanding of what it means to be healthy. PubMed, the online database of biomedical papers, accepts over 500,000 new entries each year. There are a total of 24 million. Many studies are irrelevant, esoteric, or simply confirm the conventional wisdom. Others are too small to be of value. Some of these studies, however, shake our understanding of what's "healthy" to its core.

Another reason why this matters: if we fail to accept the good news about what's bad for us, we needlessly deny ourselves pleasure. We're like the town in *Footloose* that feels guilty about dancing. Some guilty pleasures shouldn't contain a lick of guilt; we'll dig through the evidence and see why. You've probably heard the classic examples, like chocolate (packed with antioxidants) and red wine (good for the heart). These you know. But consider something that's thought of as a vice, like, say, tequila. No one has ever asked a bartender for a shot of Patrón and said, "It's good for my heart!" Yet it is. To the extent that alcohol (in moderation) confers a benefit to the heart, it doesn't really matter what you drink. Vodka. Beer. Jello shots. So if you prefer tequila to wine, take comfort that you're being just as "healthy" as the smug Pinot sippers.

Food is only one part of the story. Clever scientists, using tons of quirky experiments, have shown that "bad behavior" can have sneaky benefits. We'll meet these mavericks. One scientist in Singapore, for example, found that web surfing at work can improve productivity. The same goes for taking naps, procrastinating, and keeping a messy desk. Even gossip has its place. We think of profanity as a vice, but we'll meet a British doctor who, by measuring the physical pain of college students, found an evolutionary purpose for dropping f-bombs. Or consider the case of video games—they've been proven to sharpen our brains, quicken our reflexes, and boost our odds of staying home alone on Saturday night.

We kick ourselves for certain bad mind-sets like anger, worry, and selfishness. All of these have perks. We fear pesticides, we dread GMOs, and we're nervous about the BPAs in our plastics. But what if the science says that for all of these things—food, habits, mind-sets—the healthiest option is to simply . . . relax?

This book is meant to raise questions, challenge conventional wisdom, and knit together insights that have been previously disconnected. It is not a Complete Guide to Health. I am not a doctor. I am not a scientist. I haven't even seen that many episodes of *House.* My role is that of questioner, gatherer, and curator; my job is to explore the latest news and somehow make sense of it all. I consulted with a small army of experts from a range of disciplines—nutrition, cardiology, statistics, psychology, business, sexuality, fitness, and everything from yoga to dentistry. We'll hear from authorities like Dr. David Katz, director of the Yale University Prevention Research Center; Dr. David Tovey, the editor in chief of the Cochrane Library (a nonprofit group whose mission is to analyze health studies); Dr. David Ropeik, an expert in risk analysis, and many other doctors whose name is not David.

Whiplash: The Back-and-Forth News of Health

Monday: "Soy is bad for you!"
Tuesday: "Soy is good for you!"
Wednesday: "Fish is bad for you!"
Thursday: "Fish is good for you!"

The news of health can ping-pong back and forth, sort of the way the sheep in *Animal Farm* always agree with whoever just gave a speech. It's confusing. It's frustrating. And the experts themselves can't seem to agree. Some preach low-fat, some preach low-carb. Paleo versus plant. Non-GMO versus pro-GMO. It seems testier than Congress.

"The public is totally dismissive of health expertise," says Yale's Dr. Katz. "People see these competing headlines every day, and they conclude that we're all a pack of morons. The problem is that science doesn't work that way. You have to interpret what the study actually means, and then you have to add the new evidence to the overall weight of evidence, and then follow the direction it tips. The public doesn't know that. The media doesn't want that to happen." Katz, who was an on-air contributor for *Good Morning America* for over two years, tells me, "Frankly, they *wanted* a different dietary story each day. They didn't want to give people the same advice two weeks in a row. It's a huge problem."

So in addition to exploring the latest studies, this book has a secondary mission: creating a framework for understanding *why* the news of health can seem bipolar. It helps that we'll cover a ton of ground. We'll sprint through a broad range of topics—from coffee to nuts, milk to Q-tips—a structure that, by design, comes with its own set of bad news and good news. The bad news is that each entry is cartoonishly condensed; there's a multimillion-dollar industry in books on exercise, a topic we'll cover in three breezy pages. I've just given a taste.

The good news? Breadth has merit. By zigzagging from organic yams to the upside of naps, we can make surprising connections that are impossible in a deeper dive. In speaking with experts from so many disciplines, I found the same themes popping up again and again, sometimes word for word. This lets us build a framework. It helps us evaluate whether, for each topic, the latest study is: 1) legitimate—sometimes it is; 2) questionable—often the case; or 3) fun cocktail chatter that, in the end, is a little bit of bullshit.

I can't take credit for the roots of this framework. Much of it goes all the way back to the Greek Golden Mean, as Socrates warns us to "choose the mean and avoid the extremes on either side, as far as possible."

This leads to three key concepts: dosage, trade-offs, and absolute risk versus relative risk.

Dosage

"Courage is a virtue, but courage is a mean between cowardice and recklessness," says Dr. Barry Schwartz, author of *The Paradox of Choice*. "This principle is virtually universal. For almost everything that psychologists study—*some* of it is good, *more* of it is worse." Dosage matters. This is true in psychology, food, medicine, jogging, booze—everything. At first this seems like a simple concept, so obvious that it's not worth mentioning. But it explains so much. When a new study says that such-and-such is bad for you or good for you, it usually comes down to dosage.

Trade-Offs

Everything has a trade-off. Aspirin trims the risk of heart attacks; it might cause internal bleeding. Fish has good fatty acids; it might be poisoned with mercury. Sunshine synthesizes vitamin D on the skin; it might cause skin cancer. Bicycle commuting provides good exercise; it might lead to getting splattered by a bus.

Again, by itself, the concept is straightforward. Yet it's one reason for the seesaw-like nature of health news. Let's say something has a trade-off that's 90 percent good, 10 percent bad. (That's probably about right for fish.) The "news" might highlight the 10 percent dark side; if you're an editor at a paper or website, and if you want to keep your job, you probably won't use the accurate headline "Fish: Still Very Good for You, Despite a Probably-Not-Consequential Risk of Mercury." Instead you'll choose, "Dangerous Mercury Found in Fish!" Both headlines are technically true, but only one gives the full context. The trade-offs abound. As A. J. Jacobs says in *Drop Dead Healthy*, "I know that you should eat a lot of the Indian spice turmeric, as it fights cancer. Also that you should avoid the Indian spice turmeric, as it might contain dangerous levels of lead. One or the other."

Absolute Risk Versus Relative Risk

Let's imagine that for some wacky reason, I bought the website AliensTakeMeFirst.com. Pretend that I have a screw loose and that I really, really want to be kidnapped by aliens. So I write an impassioned essay to the little green men, insisting that if they invade Earth, they should kidnap me first. Let's also imagine that I constantly tweet about this, grow a following of other nut-jobs, and that after getting mocked on Buzzfeed, my site goes viral. It's reasonable to think that my risk of being abducted by aliens has doubled, tripled, or maybe even increased by a factor of 500 percent.

After all, if you're an alien invader and you saw my site, wouldn't you be tempted?

Stay with me here. Even though my *relative risk* has increased by a whopping 500 percent, my *absolute risk* of alien abduction is still basically 0. It went from something like 0.00000000000000000001 percent to 0.0000000000000000005 percent. True, this example sounds pretty dumb. Fair. It's a little far-fetched. Yet in virtually every facet of health—fitness, food, psychology—this dynamic is in play again and again, and it colors how we perceive risk. It's a powerful force in how the media reports health, how we read news stories, how we make choices. An example that's less goofy: pesticides in our vegetables. Yes, if we buy organic, we trim the risk from pesticides. The relative risk is lower. But what's the absolute risk in the first place? A headline might say "Pesticides Increase Risk of Some Scary Disease by 500%" but if the absolute risk is only .00001% in the first place, does it even matter? We'll explore.

This book does have one clear bias: in most of the entries, we'll focus on the "underdog research" and the counterintuitive studies. Let's take the example of stress. You already know that stress can trigger things like diabetes, heart attacks, and bigger problems like hair loss. So I'll spare us the tedium of every pro and con. Instead we'll focus on the surprising upside. This doesn't mean that stress is always good, but rather that it has certain trade-offs, and at the right dosage, we shouldn't be stressed that we're stressed. (In the case of stress, this does more than just give us peace of mind— one psychologist has a theory that *when we think of stress as a good thing*, it actually boosts our physical health.)

One quick thing. To be clear, I'm not making the case that *everything bad* is now suddenly good, and vice versa. Smokers still shouldn't smoke. Alcoholics still shouldn't drink. Please don't begin a Cheetos diet. Don't use this book as an excuse to skip the gym.

So while this book isn't anti-health, it does trace its ancestry to Woody Allen's 1973 classic, *Sleeper,* where the owner of a health store is cryogenically frozen, wakes up two hundred years later, and is revived by two futuristic doctors.

First doctor: This morning for breakfast he requested something called "wheat germ, organic honey, and tiger's milk."

Second doctor: Oh yes. Those are the charmed substances that some years ago were thought to contain life-preserving properties.

First doctor: You mean there was no deep fat? No steak or cream pies or hot fudge?

Second doctor: Those were thought to be unhealthy . . . precisely the opposite of what we now know to be true.

Like Woody, I thought all these goofy, counterintuitive studies would make a fun joke. Then I researched . . . and I found a surprising amount of truth. The stakes are real. There really *is* good news about what's bad for us. This news can make us healthier, save us money, reduce our pangs of guilt, make us happier, and improve our sex lives.*

---

*I have no idea if this last one is true, but other health books seem to claim it with no evidence, so I will, too.

And one last thing that no study can truly quantify: Steak is delicious. Bourbon is excellent. Naps are a gift from the gods. These "vices" help give life its flavor. There's living healthy and then there's *living*.

Now, finally, the science says the two are one and the same.

Let's do this.

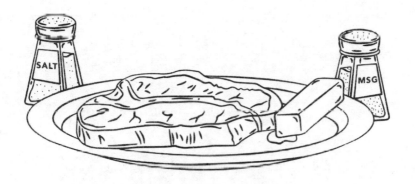

FOOD

For most of my life I was afraid of fat. Most of us are. We've had it drilled into our heads since we were toddlers: eat margarine, not butter; chicken, not beef; cereal, not eggs. Then the fear spread. We learned to fear salt, sweets, gluten, GMOs, and fast-food joints like McDonald's. How much of this is justified?

Fat

I don't remember much about what third grade taught me about nutrition, but when I close my eyes I can still visualize, in crystal-clear detail, the iconic Food Pyramid—rice, bread, and pasta toward the bottom, then juicy red steaks near the top. The message was simple and easy for children to understand: *fat makes us fat*.

We learned about the Food Pyramid around the same age we learned about things like gravity, arithmetic, and the sequence of U.S. presidents. These are basic facts. Truth with a capital

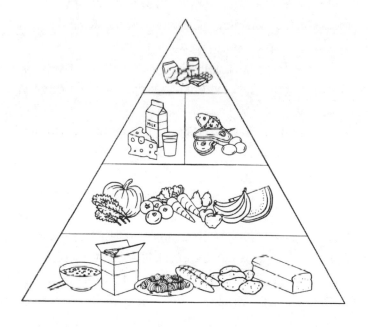

T. *George Washington was our first president. Fat is unhealthy.* For millions of Americans, the Food Pyramid is the bedrock of how we see nutrition.

Here's what third grade didn't teach us. The Food Pyramid was not, in fact, handed down to Moses by a gluten-free God. Unlike the principles of arithmetic, it has not been around for thousands or even hundreds of years. It's a recent invention. It was borne from the hypothesis—at the time a *hypothesis*, not a law—that saturated fat causes heart attacks, and since, in the 1950s, heart attacks were a national epidemic, the U.S. Department of Agriculture took drastic measures. *If saturated fat causes heart attacks, then Americans should eat more bread.*

But recently we've seen two stunning developments:

1. A review of the original 1950s-era data suggests that the premise of "saturated fat leads to heart attacks" was maybe, just maybe—or even *probably,* depending on who you ask—built on flawed studies and wobbly science. If that's actually the case, then the entire foundation of the Food Pyramid, its very reason for existence, is bunk.
2. New studies show that diets high in fat have performed just as well as, or better than, low-fat diets.

You could write an entire book about this topic, and happily, someone did just that. Nina Teicholz's *The Big Fat Surprise* is a tour de force; she spent a decade meticulously tracing every link in the scientific chain that established the doctrine of Fat=Bad, chronicling how it evolved, bit by bit, from possible theory to Law of the Land. The story is enthralling. Its tragic hero (villain?) is a man named Ancel Keys, a charismatic physiologist who, in trial after trial, spent decades trying to prove that saturated fat raises cholesterol and thus causes heart attacks. Keys was an unstoppable force. He did more to change America's diet than any one person in the twentieth century. And Teicholz argues that the foundation of his research was, well, wrong.

Let's look at a few quick highlights.

Using some "ethically questionable experiments" on schizophrenic patients in a psych ward, Keys fed some of them low-fat diets, some higher-fat. The low-fat diet led to lower levels of cholesterol and was thus considered the winner. "These experiments were hardly definitive: a series of two- to nine-week tests involving a total of only 66 people," notes Teicholz. "And Keys would soon change his mind about the findings. Nonetheless, in a style that foreshadowed how Keys would rise to the apex of the nutrition world, he promoted these tentative early results as if there were already little room for doubt. . . . This connect-the-dot exercise in 1952 was the acorn that grew into the giant oak tree of our mistrust of fat today."

Because it's tricky, and expensive, to do clinical trials of diets, Keys leaned heavily on observational studies. (In fairness, most experts do. That's often the best we've got.) He trotted all over the world to survey different cultures, seeking a link between fat consumption and heart attacks. He created a chart that would be to health what the Laffer curve is to economics—a driving force for the next sixty years of nutrition. The graph reveals a neat, tidy, step-by-step correlation for six countries high in fat and deaths due to heart disease. This seemed like a smoking gun. It seemed like the light bulb moment when we connected cigarette smoking to lung cancer. But not all scientists agreed.

As Teicholz lays it out, the "consensus" on fat was more of a 51-49 split among the researchers, with the winners writing the history books. Dr. Jacob Yerushalmy, for example, who was the founder of the biostatistics department at UC Berkeley, found that Keys' dietary graph—the lynchpin of his dietary theory—suffered from critical selection bias, as it omitted countries like Germany, Sweden, and Norway, which showed no correlation between fat and heart disease. What if you include more data? Keys' graph had six countries. Yerushalmy's had twenty-two. With this larger pool of evidence, instead of a tight correlation, it shows "only a random Jackson Pollock–like splatter of data points."

There's more. When digging through the original research, Teicholz found "one of the most stunning and troubling errors": Keys happened to sample the Cretan diet in the middle of Lent, when much of the country stops eating meat. That's one hell of a blooper. It would be like commissioning a study to gauge the amount of turkey consumed in the United States, surveying people on only one day, Thanksgiving, and then extrapolating for the rest of the year. When she confronted a surviving director of the study, he admitted, "In an ideal situation, we should not have done that. But you can't do the ideal thing all the time." Teicholz's response: "And this explanation would seem fair enough had not the Cretan data ended up being the cornerstone of our dietary advice for the past half-century."

Things quickly snowballed. Keys graced the cover of *Time*. He made buddies in the government. Despite objections from the Food and Nutrition Board of the National Academy of Sciences, the USDA would, thanks largely to Keys' hypothesis, adopt the Food Pyramid and teach it to third graders like you and me.

Phew. Let's come up for air. The point is that in those early days, plenty of scientists disagreed with Keys—offering other explanations for heart disease, like smoking—but the voices were silenced. As Keys' opponent George Mann wrote in 1978, "For a generation, research on heart disease has been more political than scientific." At a bare minimum it's *possible* that the entire Saturated Fat=Evil theory is wrong.

So what does the most current research tell us?

In the decades since all the original guesswork, study after study has failed to show a solid link between saturated fat and heart disease. They've also failed to show a link between saturated fat and obesity.

There are many examples, but let's single out the Women's Health Initiative, or WHI. This was the biggie. It had a sample size of 49,000. Launched in the early 1990s and funded by the government, it put 20,000 women on a low-fat diet (the rest were a control group) and traced the long-term impact on cholesterol. "But after a decade of eating more fruits, vegetables, and whole grains while cutting back on meat and fat, these women not only failed to lose weight, but they also did not see any significant reduction in their risk for either heart disease or cancer of any major kind," explains Teicholz. "WHI was the largest and longest trial ever of the low-fat diet, and the results indicated that the diet had quite simply failed."

Oops.

It'd be one thing if Teicholz was a lone voice in the wilderness. She's not. Way back in 2001, the Cochrane Collaboration, the unbiased, objective, nonprofit group whose mission in life is to vet health studies, reviewed all the trials on saturated fats. It concluded that "despite decades of effort and many thousands of people randomized, there is still only limited and inconclusive evidence of the effects of modification of total, saturated, mono saturated, or polyunsaturated fats on cardiovascular morbidity and mortality."

In a more recent finding, a 2014 study from Tulane showed that after a year of dieting, a low-fat diet caused women to lose 4 pounds, but a high-fat, lower-carb diet caused women to lose 8 pounds. They also had better cholesterol.

How is this possible? The real tragedy of the whole Food Pyramid, of course, is that in an effort to curb fat, we gobbled up more bread, pasta, and refined starches. And today's bread isn't our grandparents' bread. It's cheap. It spikes our insulin. It mucks up our metabolism. When we eat less fat we tend to eat more carbs— and therefore more sugar. "When insulin levels are elevated, we accumulate fat in our fat tissue; when these levels fall, we liberate fat from the fat tissue and burn it for fuel. This has been known since the early 1960s and has never been controversial," explains Gary Taubes in *Why We Get Fat*. "Our insulin levels are effectively determined by the carbohydrates we eat—not entirely, but for all intents and purposes."

Things are changing. The USDA, which once urged us to eat a low percentage of fat, no longer gives that advice. Fat is back. The Food Pyramid has been quietly removed from the USDA's nutritional guidelines, replaced with the My Plate framework that encourages a well-rounded diet. "We've given up spraying with Pam, stopped poaching, and started using salad dressing again," concludes Teicholz on a hopeful note. "Fat is the soul of flavor. Food is tasteless and cooking nearly impossible without fat."

Some of the items in this book are a bit of a wink and a joke— *feel better about your vice, but it's still a vice.* This is not one of them. There is legitimate good news about fat. Savor it.

TWO CAVEATS

1. Much of the "fat is good" theory rests upon the idea that if we eat more fat, we'll naturally eat fewer starchy carbs because we won't be as hungry. Many studies have demonstrated this. But if we take our identical diet and then, every morning, add three slices of bacon? Different story.

2. Not everyone agrees with this interpretation of Keys' work. Just as two economists can see the same unemployment report and draw two different conclusions about the Fed's policy—so many scrambled variables, so many ways to interpret the data—health experts debate the long-term changes in our health. Dr. Katz, for instance, says that the original advice from Keys was correct, but we distorted the message and never gave it a shot. "Frankly, Ancel Keys gave us perfectly good advice. He was absolutely right," Katz tells me. "But when he advised that we should eat less fat, the advice meant *eat more spinach*. The food industry said, we can't make a lot of money selling spinach, but we can invent Snackwell low-fat cookies." (He echoes the case made by Dr. Dean Ornish, who famously champions a low-fat, plant-based diet.) There are rebuttals to this rebuttal and rebuttals to those rebuttals. The debate continues.

Gluten

"People are very anti-gluten. Which bothers me, because I'm very pro-pizza," says Jimmy Kimmel in a monologue, warming up the crowd. "Some people don't eat gluten for medical reasons, and I get that . . . but a lot of people don't eat gluten because someone in their yoga class told them not to."

So he conducted a simple experiment: how many of these anti-gluten zealots actually know what gluten is? Gluten, technically, is a mix of two proteins—gliadin and glutenin. It's what gives bread its sponginess. People with celiac disease—roughly 1 percent of the population—can't digest gluten; it makes their immune system go haywire and can trigger a range of unpleasant side effects, ranging from diarrhea to death. It's worth repeating this point: 99 percent of the population does not have this problem.

In Kimmel's now-classic video, *no one knew what gluten was.* They had a vague sense that it's in bread and it's bad. At least one woman was honest. When she was asked why she avoids gluten, she laughs and says, "It makes you fat."

But here's an extra layer of irony: going gluten-free can *increase* the risk of gaining weight.

To clear up the confusion, I spoke with a longtime authority on gluten, Shelly Case, a dietician who wrote *Gluten-Free Diet: A Comprehensive Resource Guide* in 2001 and has since updated it with five editions. "Many people eventually gain weight on a gluten-free diet," she tells me. The problem is that when they create a product like gluten-free bread, in order to make the stuff edible, the manufacturer essentially swaps out the gluten with more sugars and fat. "A gluten-free bread is much more condensed and compact, and often they're not as enriched with irons and vitamins. Gluten-free does not necessarily mean healthier."

There's another complicating factor: While it's true that roughly 1 percent of the population has celiac disease, it's estimated that only 5 to 15 percent of *those people* are actually diagnosed. While 1 percent is a tiny number, 1 percent of 319 million (the U.S. population) is still over 3 million people, and if 85 percent of them are undiagnosed, that means there are at least 2 million Americans walking around with undiagnosed celiac disease. (Hence the paranoia, which, when you frame it this way, is more understandable.) But here's the catch: Case suggests that if you think you have a gluten sensitivity, *do not immediately go on a gluten-free diet.* "If they jump on the gluten-free bandwagon before they're diagnosed, the doctor won't be able to correctly diagnose them." The blood test and biopsy require gluten in the system, so going gluten-free, once again, could backfire.

When *The New Yorker*'s Michael Specter attended the Gluten and Allergen Free Expo, he encountered "gluten-free chips, gluten-free dips, gluten-free soups, and gluten-free stews; there were gluten-free breads, croutons, pretzels, and beer." He also found "a travel agent who specialized in gluten-free vacations, and a woman who helps plan gluten-free wedding receptions." After a deep dive into the issue and after consulting with the experts, Specter concludes, as I do, that it's quite possible "anti-gluten" is just the latest in a long string of misguided dietary fads that includes "low fat" and "no MSG." And fad diets fail. He ends the piece, "But I am certainly not going to live without gluten. That's just silly."

Yet it doesn't matter. Millions of people have made up their minds: gluten is evil. One study found that 30 percent of Americans think they should eat less gluten. And who can blame them? We all take our cues from nutrition experts like Miley Cyrus, who tweeted to her 18 million followers, "For everyone calling me anorexic I have a gluten and lactose allergy. It's not about weight it's about health. Gluten is crapppp anyway!"

Salt

"In spite of more than 100 years of investigations, the question of reduced sodium intake as a health prophylaxis initiative is still unsolved." These are the opening words of an analysis from the Cochrane Collaboration, the nonprofit gang of researchers who vet health studies. In 2011, they turned their gaze to salt. Or, more specifically, to low-sodium diets. They combed through 167 analyses. They crunched the numbers. They weighed all the data. The big takeaway? If you go on a low-sodium diet, this tends to result in a *1 percent decline in blood pressure.* One. Frickin'. Percent. And because most of the studies weren't equipped to gauge long-term health impacts, they glumly concluded, "we do not know if low salt diets improve or worsen health outcomes."

That's not to say that sodium isn't a problem. It can be. People who chow down on sodium tend to have higher blood pressure, which means they tend to have more heart attacks. More strokes. Higher death rates. We've known all this for some time. Then, in 2014, a study from the *New England Journal of Medicine* shook up the snow globe: Yes, it's true that people with high intakes of sodium (greater than 7 grams per day) have a higher risk of death, but people with *lower* intakes of sodium (less than 3 grams) fared even worse. Much worse. To clarify: The study showed that *the odds of a "cardiovascular event" were the highest for people who consume the* least *amount of sodium.* (Aside: I love calling a heart attack a "cardiovascular event." That's like calling the Titanic an "iceberg event.")

"Too many calories are bad for us. That doesn't mean we should consume none. Too little exercise can lead to bad outcomes. That doesn't mean you exercise to the point of hurting yourself. Too much sun can cause cancer. That doesn't mean we should never go outside," writes Dr. Aaron Carroll in an op-ed questioning why the American Heart Association gives an ultra-low recommendation of 1.5 daily grams of sodium, even though these studies show that *low sodium is more dangerous than high sodium.* Channeling the theme of this book, he adds, "It's a cliché but true: In so many things moderation is our best bet. We have to learn that when one extreme is detrimental, it doesn't mean the opposite is our safest course. It's time to acknowledge that we may be going too far with many of our recommendations."

This doesn't mean that we should immediately triple our sodium intake. But if you're not at risk of a "cardiovascular event," before you agonize over that extra pinch of salt—or scour the Internet for Fun Low-Salt Recipes!—it's worth *considering,* at least, that it's very, very, very possible that in the grand scheme of things, it just doesn't make a damn bit of difference.

Chocolate

Chocolate is the poster child of bad food that's secretly good for you. Editors have a legal obligation to run the headline "New Study: Chocolate Good for Health!" at least once a month. You've almost certainly heard about the health benefits, so we'll keep this brief.

- It can trim the risk of heart disease. It boosts your cardio-vascular system and it improves your blood flow; a 2014 study published in *Cardiovascular System* (you're

not a subscriber?) found that when people added a square
of dark chocolate to their daily diet, their blood flow
improved by 14 to 23 percent.

- It lowers blood pressure—one 2012 study suggests by an average of two to three points.

- A 2013 study found that teens who eat chocolate are thinner.

- Chocolate has something called flavonoids that trim the risk of strokes. One Swedish study showed a 17 percent lower risk for men; another showed a 20 percent lower risk for women.

- It's good for your gut. This is the focus of the latest round of research: a 2014 study found that we have certain microbes deep in our bellies, and these microbes help "ferment" the cocoa's antioxidants and its fiber.

- It might make you live longer. A 2008 Harvard study found that people who ate chocolate tended to live about a year longer than the weirdos who didn't eat chocolate. (And for the people who ate three chocolate bars a month, the risk of premature death was slashed by 36 percent.)

Why is it that the benefits are always "dark chocolate" and not just "chocolate"? Because the real benefit lies in cocoa. The lighter the chocolate, the more the cocoa has been diluted with sugar. So maybe a Hershey's bar gives you some benefit from antioxidant goodness, but it's offset by the baggage of all the refined carbs. Another theory: it's also possible that these almighty antioxidants in cocoa might not work so well with milk. As Dr. Mauro Serafini wrote in a 2013 study in *Nature*, "Our findings indicate that milk may interfere with the absorption of antioxidants from chocolate . . . and may therefore negate the potential health benefits that can be derived from eating moderate amounts of dark chocolate."

This is as good a time as any to bring up the dreaded Correlation versus Causation problem of epidemiological (or observational) studies. It's the same issue we saw with Keys—he hoped to find a link between heart disease and fat, and in some countries he might have indeed seen a link, but "link" doesn't mean causation. This problem has vexed scientists for decades. We'll see it throughout the book. In the case of chocolate, maybe it's possible that chocolate does cause people to live longer . . . but it seems more likely that people who eat chocolate tend to have more income, and therefore better access to health care.

For any health study, the most bulletproof evidence is a randomly assigned clinical trial, where, for example, group A takes a drug, group B takes a sugar pill as a placebo. This is ideal. This is rare. Instead, researchers hunt for patterns and hope to tease out insights from large populations, hoping we can *infer* causation. Sometimes this is reasonable and sometimes it's not. As one critic of correlation-causation noted, athletes on basketball teams tend to be taller than athletes not on basketball teams; this does not mean that if you join the basketball team, you will get taller.

Or my favorite example: in the 1980s, when analyzing crime in New York City, one researcher found a link between the sale of ice-cream-makers and the rate of violent sexual crimes. One takeaway is that we should banish the sale of ice-cream makers. Another takeaway is that there's a confounding variable, *heat*, and that crime tends to rise in the summer, which is also when people eat ice cream.

GMOs

Genetically Modified Organism. The words make us squirm. They're ugly. We visualize things like blue tomatoes, square watermelons, or men with three arms. GMOs sound unhealthy. Unproven. Unsafe.

This is why thousands of angry citizens march in protest against Monsanto, the Darth Vader of GMO corporations, a company that, in one poll, is the third most hated company on the planet. In one protest, adorable little children held up cardboard signs that said "We are not science experiments."

Should companies be forced to label their cyberfood as GMOs? This holy war is very much in flux. There are two simple facts, however, that we can't really escape:

1. Most of us already eat a diet that's heavy in GMOs. (We just don't think about it.)
2. Virtually all the mainstream science, in study after study, has concluded that GMOs are as healthy as non-GMOs.

As Molly Ball writes in *The Atlantic*, "No widely accepted science supports the idea that GMOs are inherently dangerous to people's health or the environment." Ninety percent of the corn, cotton, and soybeans planted in the United States is *already* genetically modified. The World Health Organization and the American Medical Association have both given GMOs the official thumbs-up.

This creates a political role reversal. "Scientists, who have come to rely on liberals in political battles over stem-cell research, climate change, and the teaching of evolution, have been dismayed to find themselves at odds with their traditional allies on this issue," writes Amy Harmon in *The New York Times*. "Some compare the hostility to GMOs to the rejection of climate-change science, except with liberal opponents instead of conservative ones." Exhibit A: Self-described "lifelong environmentalist" Mark Lynas, a Cornell University researcher who has written two books on climate change. In 2015 he wrote an op-ed, "How I Got Converted to GMO Food," noting that while only 37 percent of the public thinks it's safe to eat GMOs, with scientists it's 88 percent. "I decided I could no longer continue taking a pro-science position on global warming and an anti-science position on G.M.O.s," explains Lynas. "There is an equivalent level of scientific consensus on both issues, I realized, that climate change is real and genetically modified foods are safe. I could not defend the expert consensus on one issue while opposing it on the other."

You could make a compelling case that GMOs are actually *better* for the environment. With genetic modification, farmers can plant seeds that are, by design, resistant to certain insects. Since these new seeds won't be eaten by bugs, this means we can spray less insecticide. We kill fewer insects. It's cleaner.

"It doesn't make any sense," Dr. Alison Van Eenennaam, an expert in animal genomics and biotechnology at UC Davis, tells me over the phone. "There are hundreds of peer-reviewed studies showing that they are no different. That's what the data shows."

It's hard for data to trump emotion, and most of us are emotional about our food. It doesn't *feel* right for scientists to use computers to program food, but then again, haven't we been doing this, to some extent, since farmers made "garden varieties" of plants, or, arguably, since Columbus brought pineapples to England?

The big counter to all of this, of course, is that maybe *we just don't know*. What if there are long-term effects of GMOs that we can't anticipate? What if there's some sneaky danger to the environment that escapes all these hundreds of studies? To paraphrase Donald Rumsfeld, there are the known unknowns and then there are the unknown unknowns.

"You can always say, 'But what about in fifty years?' Well, what do we know about *anything* in fifty years? We want zero risk, but we're quite prepared to accept risk in every other walk of life," Van Eenennaam tells me.

Then she gives me a bit of a riddle. "Who's the main consumer of GMOs?"

"Um . . ." I sense I'm falling into a trap.

"Animals," she says. "Over 90 percent of the corn in the United States is genetically engineered, and the major thing we do with the soybean and corn, of course, is to use it for animal feed."

"Right."

"We consume nine billion chickens every year. That's more than there are people on Earth. We're already eating a diet that's almost entirely genetically engineered."

And then she told me about her research that had not yet been made public. Since chickens, steers, and the like tend to live such short (and miserable) lives, there are now many generations of livestock that were raised on a GMO-heavy diet. This gives us a massive dataset. She crunched the numbers on a population that includes over 100 billion livestock and found no differences in mortality rates. This suggests that in generation after generation, the GMOs have no impact. The chickens also had an improved feed-to-grain ratio, indicating they stayed healthy. "I challenge anyone else to show me a dataset with a 100 billion observations."

THE COUNTER

So is it fair to call anti-GMOers anti-science? Maybe, maybe not. After acknowledging that the scientific consensus *does* say that GMOs are safe to eat, Tamar Haspel suggests a compromise in the *Washington Post*. "Most GMO opponents aren't anti-science; they're anti-GMO, and therefore see the large body of science that contradicts their ideas as tainted by association with industry, flawed methodologically, done by biased scientists or otherwise dismissible. They are, in fact, pro-science—toward science that confirms their beliefs. (GMO supporters, and humans in general, are just as susceptible to this kind of confirmation bias.)"

There's also the economic argument: many make the case that GMOs and Monsanto, ultimately, squeeze the local farmer.

McDonald's

McDonald's takes a lot of shit, and rightly so: much of the food is crap. But was the *Super Size Me* gimmick really fair? The dude ate the equivalent of *ten Big Macs a day*. And he got fat. Shocker.

Here's a different perspective. In 2014, a fifty-four-year-old science teacher named John Cisna also went on the McDonald's diet, but instead of pigging out with burgers, he capped himself at 2,000 calories a day. For six months he ate nothing but McDonald's.

The results?

- He lost 61 pounds.
- He shaved his body mass index from 38 to 30.

- His cholesterol plunged from 249 to 190.
- He even cashed in by writing the book *My McDonald's Diet*, detailing how he created meals from their menu of salads, egg whites, and bowls of maple oatmeal.

"Many people blame McDonald's and other fast-food restaurants for the country's obesity epidemic," explains Cisna in his book. "I never fully bought into the myth that burger joints were ruining the country. As a scientist I thought *Super Size Me* was irresponsible journalism. . . . Of course someone who purposely eats 5,000 calories a day with no exercise is going to gain weight. What's the big surprise here?"

True, this science teacher, who lives in Iowa, is in a very different place than a low-income mother who's trying to feed her kids, using greasy burgers from the dollar menu to make ends meet. There's a legitimate policy debate to be had. Too often, though, we use the Golden Arches—or Taco Bell, Burger King, or Pizza Hut—as a scapegoat. They're easy targets.

Neither of these extreme diets is fair. McDonald's is not a miracle diet. McDonald's is not the reason we're fat. McDonald's is just food. Some good, some bad. What we do with it is up to us.

We'll have plenty more to say about food—eggs, bacon, carbs, even candy—but let's take a break for cocktails.

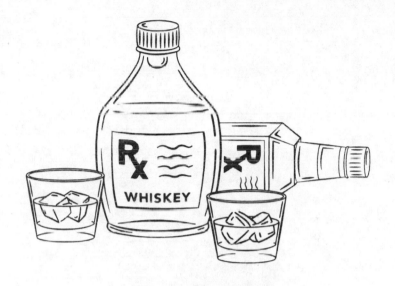

DRINK

Alcohol may be man's worst enemy, but the Bible says love your enemy.—Frank Sinatra

Whiskey

A bourbon a day keeps the doctor away. Actually, that might be understating it: whiskey can save your life. And it might be healthier to drink three a day than one a day. No, really.

It doesn't have any carbs. The average serving has fewer than 70 calories, zero cholesterol, and zero grams of sugar and sodium. It might even be healthier than red wine. "Research has shown that there are even greater health benefits to people who drink single-malt whiskies. Why? Single-malt whiskies have more ellagic acid than red wine," explained Dr. Jim Swan, unveiling a 2005 study suggesting that ellagic acid, which comes from barley, seeks out and destroys rogue cells. "Whiskey can protect you from cancer and science proves it."

Others in the medical community quickly pointed out that "ellagic acid" is also found in raspberries, strawberries, plants, pecans, and lots of food that doesn't get you shitfaced. It's also possible that the study was backed by the whiskey industry. But still. Even if you don't totally buy the ellagic acid argument, whiskey does have one important ingredient that has a real health benefit: alcohol.

In one of the happiest quirks of humanity, alcohol confers a variety of benefits *regardless of its form*, whether it's a fine merlot or a shot of Jägermeister. "There really isn't any evidence that one is better than the other," says Dr. David Hanson, who sometimes pops up on CNN and NBC as an "alcohol expert." He explains that out of any ten random studies of alcohol, some might say that red wine is the healthiest, some say beer, some say spirits. "The reason is that the primary beneficial element of alcohol beverages is . . . alcohol."

Alcohol improves our blood. It trims bad cholesterol and boosts the good stuff, reducing the risk of clotting. This can help our heart. Study after study has shown that when people drink alcohol, compared to those who abstain, the rates of cardiovascular disease are lower by 20 to 50 percent. It can fight diabetes and dementia. Again and again, bewildered scientists have shown that drinkers tend to live longer.

There are ten thousand asterisks to all this, of course. The first: just as we saw with chocolate, maybe these studies jumble correlation and causation? Critics cite the problem of selection bias, arguing that people who drink in moderation, in general, tend to be healthier and more prone to exercise. To isolate this variable, scientists in Denmark studied the longevity of twelve thousand people to explore the interplay of booze and exercise. They looked at four groups: people who

Exercised and drank moderately
Exercised and didn't drink
Didn't exercise and drank moderately
Didn't exercise and didn't drink

The unhealthiest group (defined by the shortest life span) was the one that didn't exercise and didn't drink. The healthiest? Exercised and drank moderately. Exercisers who drank were healthier than exercisers who didn't drink.

Next asterisk: Wait, but what about those studies that show that even moderate drinking, for women, can increase the risk of breast cancer? This is also true. Alcohol giveth and alcohol taketh away. Yet another trade-off. So how does this square with alcohol helping you live longer? As Hanson explains it, compared to heart disease, relatively fewer women die of breast cancer—roughly 5 percent. "So if you increase your chance of breast cancer by 10 percent, your overall chance of dying from it hasn't increased very much." Back to that concept of *absolute risk*. On the other hand, the logic goes, if you drink whiskey in moderation, you could reduce the chances of cardiovascular disease—a more likely cause of death, a higher absolute risk—by a third. "It's a no-brainer, really," says Hanson. "If you're concerned about all causes of mortality, the math is pretty straightforward." (Context matters. This might not be true for, say, a young woman with a healthy heart and a family history of breast cancer.)

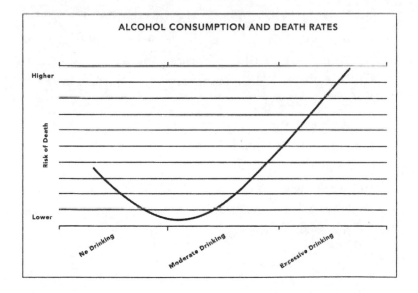

ALCOHOL CONSUMPTION AND DEATH RATES

These studies suggest that mortality rates and booze have a J-shaped curve. Nondrinkers have a higher early-death rate than moderate drinkers, but once we drink too much, the thirty-seven thousand problems with excessive drinking (poisoned livers, anemia, heart attacks, depression, high blood pressure, nerve damage, depression, drunk driving, acting like an ass-hat) outweigh the benefit.

Hanson isn't just some rogue doctor who's bucking the trend. In 2008, a study by the Research Society on Alcoholism found that "a considerable body of epidemiology associates moderate alcohol consumption with significantly reduced risks of coronary heart disease and, albeit currently a less robust relationship, cerebrovascular (ischemic) stroke." Hundreds of studies have shown this. As Yale's Dr. David Katz told me point-blank, "I don't think there is a debate. It's very clear mechanistically, in both observational and in interventionist trials, that moderate alcohol intake reduces cardiovascular risk factors and cardiovascular disease."

So what's "moderate" drinking, anyway? The official guidelines are two drinks a day for men and one for women, although some studies have shown that to optimize its impact against cardiovascular disease, the right amount could be as much as *five*. (I'm skeptical.) "In these studies, people have a tendency to underreport how much they drink—with some exceptions, like guys in fraternities—so my guess is that the real number is higher than we think," says Hanson.

This is why, when you walk into a dive bar at 2:00 a.m. and see all those old men slouched over their whiskeys, they are the healthiest people you will ever see.

Coffee

We have a curious relationship with coffee. We drink it, we crave it, we love it. In the United States alone, every day we drink a collective 400 million cups—more cups than total people—yet for some reason we feel guilty. We view coffee as a necessary evil, a bad habit, a shameful crutch. There's a nagging sense that we're doing something unhealthy to our bodies, unnatural, and that eventually we'll have to pay the piper.

Just as we saw with fat, it's time to shed the guilt.

"Trying to quit coffee" makes as much sense as "trying to quit broccoli." There are good drugs and bad drugs, and caffeine wears a White Hat. When caffeine enters the bloodstream, it worms its way into the brain and blocks something called adenosine, and this unleashes extra bits of dopamine. Caffeine lights up the neurons. In study after study, coffee boosts our memory, reaction times, mood, and our ability to stay awake through the regional sales meeting.

It saves lives. In Australia, for example, scientists studied the patterns of a thousand truck drivers and found that even when you hold other variables constant, the coffee-drinking truckers were 63 percent less likely to crash. Other studies have linked coffee to a reduction in oral cancers, a lower risk of type 2 diabetes, and stronger livers. Studies with athletes have shown a boost to physical performance, often in the neighborhood of 11 percent. And while the most obvious ingredient of coffee is caffeine, it also provides B2, B5, potassium, and magnesium.

Not only does coffee make us sharper *in the moment*, it might even improve our memories *in the long run*. In a 2013 study at John

Hopkins, researchers showed several pictures to a group of one hundred people. One panel was given caffeine, one panel no caffeine, and one panel a placebo. (This is a good study.) The next day, the scientists showed the volunteers another round of pictures, and they asked them to remember if they were the same, different, or similar to the original batch. The caffeine consumers had the best recall.

Or if you want to get a little morbid, one study found that coffee drinkers are less likely to jump off a bridge. In 2012, when Harvard researchers analyzed data from two hundred thousand adults, they concluded that people who drink two to four cups a day were 50 percent less likely to kill themselves. (I'm skeptical that there are enough suicides to make this statistically significant. But still.)

And in the final analysis, coffee drinkers tend to flat-out live longer. In 2012, researchers analyzed the mortality patterns of over four hundred thousand people. Once they controlled for variables like age, exercise, and diet, they found that for those who drank three cups per day, the risk of dying decreased by 10 percent. "It's a modest effect," said lead researcher Dr. Neal D. Freedman. "But the biggest concern for a long time has been that drinking coffee is a risky thing to do. . . . Although we cannot infer a causal relationship between coffee drinking and lower risk of death, we believe these results do provide some reassurance that coffee drinking does not adversely affect health."

The normal asterisks apply: some of these studies blur correlation with causation, too much coffee is bad for you, and far too much can kill you. Dosage, dosage, dosage.* And caffeine sensi-

---

* But this is true of everything, including water.

tivity can vary dramatically from person to person. My father, for instance, is so caffeine-sensitive that a chocolate chip cookie will give him insomnia.

Wait, but isn't too much coffee bad for your heart? Maybe in excess. But in the last few years, the scientific community has debunked the idea that coffee is linked to cardiovascular disease. "Recent studies have generally found no connection between coffee and an increased risk of cancer or heart disease," advises the Mayo Clinic, concluding, "For most people, the health benefits outweigh the risks."

Of course I'm biased. If you told me that coffee was *certain* to reduce my life by five years, I'm still not sure I'd give it up. The fact that this is exactly the same kind of logic a drug addict uses when describing heroin is totally irrelevant.

WHY ARE THERE SO MANY HEALTH STUDIES?

In the time it takes you to read this book, hundreds—if not thousands—of health studies will go to press. Thank (or blame) that old chestnut of academia: *Publish or perish.* "The way that science is incentivized, and the way that professors get tenure, leads to these discrete little one-nutrient studies that, often, don't really tell us much about anything," says Dr. Ivan Oransky, one of those awe-inspiring multitaskers who's somehow a professor of medical journalism at NYU, the Editorial Director of MedPageToday.com, and the founder of RetractionWatch.com.

"In science you have what's referred to as the 'Least Publishable Unit,' or LPU. It's also called 'salami slicing,'" Oransky tells me. "The idea is that you slice everything narrow enough so that you can get a paper out of it, but it doesn't taste very good. It's just a thin slice of salami. You can't get a sandwich out of it."

Take our example of coffee. Conducting a proper study of "Is coffee good for you?" would be a sprawling, costly, time-consuming trial with hundreds of variables and years of data. "You need to publish. Yes, you would certainly get tenure if you're the first author of that massive study, but you'd get that tenure when you're 7,000 years old," he says, laughing. Instead, researchers are motivated to tackle "the *bare minimum* of what's publishable, and no more than that."

So instead of the study we all really want—"Is coffee good for you?"—the LPU, or Least Publishable Unit, churns out papers like *How Does Coffee Impact People with Liver Cancer?* The scope is narrow. And it leaves plenty of room for follow-up studies, like how coffee impacts the pancreas, or pregnancies, or our short-term memory. They can't make a global Thumbs-Up or Thumbs-Down. This isn't to knock the brilliant scientists and researchers who dedicate their careers to advancing knowledge—we need them. We owe them. But it does help explain, though, why we always see more articles, more back-and-forth, and more WTF.

Beer

Beer is packed with a nutrient called silicon, which can help strengthen our bones. (Your move, milk.) Scientists from UC Davis analyzed the brewing process of a hundred different beers, finding that the average has 30 milligrams of silicon per liter, with beers heavy on barley and hops, such as IPAs, providing the biggest bang for the buck. "Choose the beer you enjoy. Drink it in moderation. It is contributing silicon (and more) to your good health," said Dr. Charles Bamforth, the study's lead researcher. Beer is rich in vitamin B and fiber. Thanks to its high water content, it can trim our risk of getting kidney stones by 40 percent, according to a Finnish study.

And maybe it can make us smarter. "Low levels of alcohol appear to have cognitive benefits," concluded Dr. Francine Grodstein, after a 2005 study of the long-term impact of moderate drinking on cognitive functions, especially for the elderly. "Women who consistently were drinking about one-half to one drink per day had both less cognitive impairment as well as less decline in their cognitive function compared to women who didn't drink at all." Grodstein's team analyzed the data collected on twelve thousand nurses between the ages of seventy and eighty—you know, the typical beer guzzlers—and found a long-term link between moderate drinking and improved memory. When these elderly nurses consumed one drink a day over a four-year period, the chances of mental degradation declined by around 15 to 20 percent. "On average, women who drank moderately tended to have the memory and reasoning agility of someone about a year and a half younger than those who abstained," *The Washington Post* reported. This is why on the nights you drink beer, you always seem to make extra smart decisions.*

---

* Sadly, there's something else beer is rich in: carbs. Another trade-off. If you're drinking a steady diet of beer, the carbs make it that much harder to drop weight.

Drinking During Pregnancy

As a man who is not a doctor, I feel uniquely qualified to give advice on whether it's healthy to drink alcohol while pregnant. The conventional wisdom, as everyone knows, is along the lines of what the Mayo Clinic suggests:

> One drink isn't likely to hurt your baby, but no level of alcohol has been proved safe during pregnancy. The safest bet is to avoid alcohol entirely. Consider the risks. Mothers who drink alcohol have a higher risk of miscarriage and stillbirth. Too much alcohol during pregnancy can result in fetal alcohol syndrome, which can cause facial deformities, heart defects and mental retardation. Even moderate drinking can impact your baby's brain development.

Let's let those words sink in: "your *baby's brain development.*" With the stakes so high and the upside so low, who wants to toss the dice? It's a line that no one wants to cross—not mothers, not doctors, not most academics. No politician will ever get elected on a platform of "Let Pregnant Women DRINK!" The Centers for Disease Control is more blunt: "There is no safe time to drink alcohol during pregnancy . . . .When a pregnant woman drinks alcohol, so does her baby."

But it's also true that the experts themselves don't fully agree. In 2010, roughly eight hundred obstetricians were surveyed as to whether it's okay for pregnant women to drink alcohol. As Emily Oster, author of *Expecting Better: Why the Conventional Pregnancy Wisdom Is Wrong,* noted at the time, "Sixty percent of the OBs said none, but the other 40 percent said some alcohol was fine." The standards in Europe and the UK are more lax, with the British government's official guidelines sanctioning one to two drinks per week.

Doctors and the media are (understandably) gun-shy about trumpeting these findings, but some studies find no correlation between moderate alcohol consumption and complications with babies. Zilch. "There appears to be no increased risk of negative impacts of light drinking in pregnancy on behavioral or cognitive development in seven-year-old children," concluded Professor Yvonne Kelly of the University College, London, who, in 2013, codirected a study of ten thousand kids. Her team tested the kids' cognitive abilities and then split them into groups based on whether the mother drank lightly during pregnancy (one to two drinks per week) or abstained completely. They found no difference.

Other studies found the same thing. One analysis from the University of Copenhagen, which combed through the survey results of thirty-seven thousand women, found something even more blasphemous: the moderate drinkers tended to be associated with kids who had *better* mental health.* (WARNING: Correlation versus Causation Alert. The women who drank occasionally were also more likely to go to the gym and have a higher income. Don't take this study to the bank.) Even the study's coauthor, researcher Janni Niclasen, seemed taken aback by the results and almost apologized for them. "I really think we should recommend abstaining during pregnancy. I really believe that even a glass of wine now and again is really damaging."

Every doctor agrees that drinking *heavily* is profoundly damaging to the fetus. And every doctor agrees that drinking *nothing* is guaranteed to be the safest. But surely every doctor would also agree that one microscopic drop of alcohol isn't going to poison the fetus. Two drops? Three? On a continuum, where do we draw the line between one drop and four glasses? What dosage? This is hard to test and quantify, since, for obvious ethical reasons, we can't do a controlled clinical trial where some pregnant women are asked to hit the bottle. We have to rely on messy observational studies, each polluted with so many other variables. And while some studies show no harm, others do, such as a 2011 Danish study that found that "even low amounts of alcohol consumption during early pregnancy increased the risk of spontaneous abortion substantially. The results indicate that the fetus is particularly susceptible to alcohol exposure early in pregnancy."

In *Expecting Better*, Emily Oster summarizes these studies and concludes that "based on this data, many women may feel comfortable with an occasional glass of wine—even up to one a day—in later trimesters. (More caution in the first trimester—no more than two drinks a week—because of some evidence of miscarriage risk.)"

The backlash was swift. Even before her book hit shelves, the National Organization on Fetal Alcohol Syndrome unleashed a scathing press release that challenged Oster's "deeply flawed and harmful advice." As she describes in *Slate*, some Amazon reviewers called her an alcoholic, with one chiding, "Emily Oster claims that her 2-year-old daughter is perfectly healthy, yet the full impact of the alcohol exposure on her child will not be evident until the adolescent years." Ouch. So it's a bit of a touchy subject.

(Speaking of . . . Did I mention that I AM NOT A DOCTOR, and if you are a pregnant woman, please do not shout "Whoooo hoooooo!" and sprint to the nearest pub.)

Tequila

Some history: tequila is made from a plant called agave. These plants grow like wild in the hills of Mexico, which is why the best tequilas tend to have names like Don Julio, Cuervo, and Patrón. A natural sugar, called agavin, comes from this plant, and according to scientists in Mexico, agavin has properties that might just help us lose weight and fight diabetes.

The researchers studied two different groups of mice: one group ate and drank as normal, and the other had its water spiked with agavins. The agavin-drinking mice had higher glucose levels; they tended to eat less, and their bodies produced more insulin. The agavins acted as an appetite suppressant. (In an unrelated experiment, I, too, have found that when I drink lots of tequila, I rarely think of food.) "We believe agavins have a great potential as a light sweetener," wrote the director of the study, Dr. Mercedes G. López. "They are . . . highly soluble, with a low glycemic index and a neutral taste. . . . This puts agavins in a tremendous position for their consumption by obese and diabetic people." Who wants to join me on a tequila diet?

And yet another benefit of alcohol in general: creativity. "Write drunk, edit sober," said Hemingway.* Now we have the data to back this up. In the earlier study from the beer section (with the elderly nurses), scientists suggested that alcohol could have a long-term effect on halting cognitive decline, but they didn't evaluate

---

*Let's ignore, for the moment, that 1) There's some doubt on whether he actually said this; and 2) Hemingway was an alcoholic who stuffed a shotgun in his mouth and pulled the trigger.

whether it makes us smarter in the moment. A more recent study did just that. Researchers from the University of Illinois rounded up forty men, gave half of them two drinks, and then conducted a series of mental tests. Not surprisingly, when it came to the ability to focus, the drinkers didn't perform as well. But then it gets interesting. They also created a bar game: the men were given three words and then had to think of a fourth to fit the pattern. The drinkers successfully completed 40 percent more of the puzzles than the nondrinkers—and faster. "We have this assumption that being able to focus on one part of a problem or having a lot of expertise is better for problem solving," said the lead researcher, Dr. Jennifer Wiley. "But that's not necessarily true. Innovation may happen when people are not so focused. Sometimes it's good to be distracted."

In a word: *shots*!

Red Wine

Yawn. I know, I know, you've heard this one before: 97 percent of dinner parties include that guy who says, winking, as if he's sharing a naughty secret, "Red wine is good for the heart."

We laugh and we drink but we don't *really* believe this. It feels like an old wives' tale, a joke, a rationale for uncorking that second bottle. And even *if* red wine might be good for your heart, it's still *alcohol*, which means it's a vice and therefore bad for us, right?

Not according to Hippocrates. "It is better to be full of drink than full of food," wrote the father of western medicine, who, frankly, is probably overstating the case. He used wine for fevers, wounds, and everything from cleaning babies to treating diarrhea.

Just like all forms of alcohol, red wine fights bad cholesterol, thins the blood, unclogs our arteries, helps the heart, and makes it 74 percent easier to get through an awkward first date. But on top of these benefits, red wine has an antioxidant called resveratrol, which comes from the seeds of red grapes. It might do wonders. A scientist at Johns Hopkins, for example, suggested that resveratrol could help protect our brain in the event of a stroke. He fed some mice a bit of resveratrol, and a control group none. Then, to induce strokes, he cut off blood to the mice's brains. (Here I'm imagining evil maniacal laughter.) The resveratrol mice had less brain damage.

Other studies have linked red wine to a lower risk of prostate cancer, an improved resistance to insulin (which trims the risk of diabetes), and better odds of avoiding dementia. And while there *is* generally a link between most alcohol and a heightened risk of breast cancer, red wine—thanks, once again, to resveratrol—might have the opposite effect, as it lowers estrogen levels and increases testosterone. *Red wine increases testosterone.* (New slogan for the wine industry: "Act like a man and drink merlot.")

One serious rap on alcohol—besides alcoholism, drunk driving, and acting like a tool—is that it's bad for your liver. Red wine could be the exception. "Modest wine consumption may not only be safe for the liver but may actually decrease the prevalence of NAFLD (non-alcoholic fatty liver disease)," said Dr. Jeffrey Schwimmer of UC San Diego School of Medicine, who led the study. "The odds of having suspected NAFLD . . . was reduced by 50 percent in individuals who drank one glass of wine a day." So while there's no crystal clear verdict on whether it's healthier to drink wine, beer, or spirits, wine ~~snobs~~ enthusiasts have plenty of ammo.

Counterargument: some argue that the resveratrol claims of red wine are exaggerated. "I identified this claim as bullshit from the start," writes psychiatrist and addiction expert Dr. Stanton Peele in *Pacific Standard*, citing a different study that showed there was *not* a link between resveratrol and a healthier heart. "It was simply a way to avoid recognizing that alcohol is good for you by claiming instead that alcohol's benefits are due to some other ingredient."

We'll let Hippocrates have the final word: "Wine is the best product of humanity, because it can be drunk in good and bad health too, but of course moderately." (Then again, he was also a fan of burning patients with hot copper rods. No doctor is perfect.)

Vodka, Cognac, Gin, Moonshine, and Every Other Form of Alcohol

The downsides of excessive alcohol are so tragic that, understandably, the health world is skittish about encouraging us to drink.

But is that the right thing to do? If you poll a hundred random people on the street and ask them, "What's healthier: drinking alcohol or abstaining?" my guess is that 80 percent would say it's healthier to abstain. If you believe most of these studies, however—and many doctors do—that's just not the case. Heart disease remains the number one cause of death, and alcohol is good for the heart.

How much of our attitude about alcohol is driven by hard science, and how much comes from a culture that still has roots in the temperance movement? In his manifesto "The Truth We Won't Admit: Drinking Is Healthy," Peele argues that "the evidence that abstinence from alcohol is a cause of heart disease and early death is irrefutable—yet this is almost unmentionable in the United States. Even as health bodies like the CDC and *Dietary Guidelines for Americans* (prepared by Health and Human Services) now recognize the decisive benefits from moderate drinking, each such announcement is met by an onslaught of opposition and criticism, and is always at risk of being reversed."

This doesn't condone binge drinking. This doesn't let abusers off the hook. And this varies from person to person. But Peele notes that if a celebrity died from lung cancer, the obituary would surely mention that he's a smoker. But if he died from heart attack, "no one would dare suggest that quitting drinking might be responsible for his heart attack." Peele reminds us of a classic anecdote: In 2000, David Letterman had quintuple bypass surgery; he later invited Bryant Gumbel on his show as a guest. Letterman had given up booze many years before. Gumbel had not. Letterman had given up cigars. Gumbel had not. Letterman is lean and trim. Gumbel is not. Letterman asked him, "How come I do everything healthy and you smoke cigars and drink and I end up on the surgery table?"

So if you're an alcoholic or at risk of being an alcoholic, don't drink. If you can't drink responsibly, don't drink. If you choose not to drink for religious or moral or personal reasons, don't drink. If you are Lindsay Lohan, don't drink.

But if you're not drinking because you think it's unhealthy or, more likely, you *do* drink in moderation but you feel kinda guilty about it . . . relaaaax. Next round's on me.

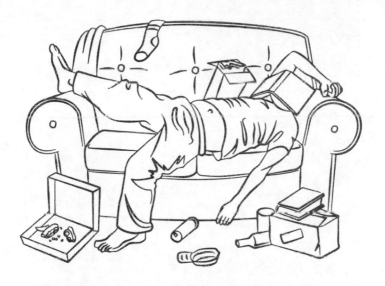

BAD HABITS

Just as we feel guilty about "bad food" and "bad drinks," we tend to regret bad habits. They embarrass us. Maybe we keep a messy desk, take naps, gossip, or wait until the last minute to get work done. Maybe we complain too much. Cuss too much.

All of this could be good for us.

Profanity

Britain. 2007. It started with a woman giving birth. As the doctor told her to *push-push-push!* she screamed in pain and yelled a blast of obscenities.

Her husband watched, fascinated. This woman could really cuss.

"Is this normal?" he asked the midwife, half-joking.

"Don't be embarrassed. It's a perfectly normal part of giving birth," the midwife told him.

Hmmmm. This got him thinking. He happened to be a scientist, Dr. Richard Stephens, and as he told me years later, "The delivery of the baby was the starting point. In this perfectly rapturous, beautiful moment of giving birth, she's cursing like a sailor."

Why would his wife start dropping f-bombs? And if it's a "perfectly normal" part of going into labor, why does everyone do it? What's the root cause? Logically, Stephens reasoned, there must be a biological purpose for profanity. "Swearing is obviously useful; if it wasn't useful, people wouldn't do it," he tells me. "We only do things that give us rewards or benefits; that's just the way the world is."

So he dedicated his work to proving that swearing can, in fact, give us measurable benefits. In a delightfully oddball experiment, he had a group of student volunteers dunk their hands into a tub of freezing water. He measured how long they could keep their hands in the ice water. (Stephens sounds like a gentle man with a lovely British accent, but the experiment, we must admit, does seem a touch sadistic.) He split the poor bastards into two groups:

Group A) While holding their hands in the freezing water, they said their favorite swear word over and over again, like a woman in labor.

Group B) While holding their hands in the freezing water, they said a neutral word over and over again, like "toothbrush" or "applesauce."

Group A, the f-bombers, reported experiencing less pain. They were able to keep their hands under water 40 seconds longer than group B—roughly *twice* as long.

So how does this work? One theory is that taboo words are, inherently, more loaded with emotion than neutral words, and that they tap into a different chunk of the brain. "There's indirect evidence that swearing isn't associated with the cortex—where most language is—but instead taps into the deeper parts of the brain structure," says Stephens. Profanity, therefore, is able to trigger our flight-or-fight mechanism, which can unleash adrenaline to help us tolerate pain or squeeze out a baby.

To buttress the theory that profanity is an emotional language, he then conducted an experiment to see whether our *fluency* with profanity changes in different emotional states. He recruited another batch of college volunteers. This time they played video games for ten minutes: one group played video golf, another played a violent first-person shooter. After the gaming, each student took a "swearing fluency test," where you have one minute to write down as many swear words as you can. The control group (the golfers) only recorded seven, but the first-person shooters recorded eight. "That doesn't sound like much," admits Stephens, "But it's statistically significant. In psychology, the difference between seven and eight is night and day."

Of course I needed to know more about this swearing fluency test, which is clearly the best test ever. "People only got *seven*?" I ask. "That seems really low."

"It's harder than you think. People usually get five or six pretty easily, and then it really trails off."

"What counts as a swear word?"

"You can say fuck or fuck-face or fucking, but that's just a variation of fuck," says Stephens in his pleasant English accent—this was easily the highlight of my research. "So fuck-face gets one point, but you can't look around the room and say fuck-table."

Afterward I took my own swearing fluency test. I was sure I could pump out at least twenty, maybe thirty. I am not good at many things in life, but swearing is one of them.

My score? Ten. I was so disappointed. But Stephens was right: it really is harder when you remove variants from the equation. For example, in my mind, an *ass*-clown is a harmless buffoon, whereas an ass bag is more of a dick. (Go ahead and take the swearing fluency test for yourself—it's a fun 60 seconds.)

The point is that our ability to use profanity is linked to our emotional state, an observation that squares with a 2011 experiment conducted by the University of Bristol, which found that it's the *swear words themselves*, and not their meaning, that triggers an emotional response. The study hooked up volunteers to a machine that measured sweat levels, which is a proxy for measuring stress, and then asked them to say either actual swear words or their euphemisms.

People felt more stress when they said the taboo words . . . even when the meanings are identical. (In other words, your stress levels are higher when you say "Fuck" than when you say "Fiddle-sticks.") Taboo words have power. So while we roll our eyes at people who say "Oh, sugar!" instead of "Oh, shit!" there actually is a measurable, physiological difference in how the words are felt.

Or let's take the most provocative and controversial word you know. Yeah, that one. In his stand-up act *Chewed Up*, Louis CK mocks TV reporters for going on air and saying "the N-word," because we all know what that awful word means, and instead of using the euphemism, says Louis, you might as well just man up and say the awful word, because otherwise, you're forcing *the listener* to fill in the blanks and say the actual N-word in our heads. I adore Louis and it's a clever argument, but since the *taboo words themselves* trigger more of an emotional impact than the meaning behind that taboo, in this case he might be mistaken. If I actually printed the N-word (which I will not do) you will physically feel worse than you do this second. For good or evil, substitute words just don't pack the same punch.

Back to the benefits of swearing: it can help your career. "Profanity in the workplace can be a morale booster and inspire a sense of team spirit," concludes a 2007 study from the University of East Anglia, as it can loosen us up and help break the ice. Then again . . . one person's "loosening up" is another person's "hostile work environment." Just ask the former CEO of Yahoo, Carol Bartz, who once grumbled to Yahoo investors that there's "nobody fucking doing anything" and once threatened her employees that she would "drop-kick them to fucking Mars." After an ugly split with Yahoo she later said she regretted the profanity.

Too much profanity can dilute the impact. Another one of Stephens's experiments found that "the higher the swearing frequency, the less was the benefit for pain tolerance." If you abuse it you lose it.

So just like everything in this book, of course, it comes down to fucking moderation.

Messiness

The logic is familiar to every seven-year-old: *Why do I have to make my bed if it's just going to get messy again?*

Eventually we surrender. As we learn to make our beds and do our chores, we grow up to embrace, and even fetishize, the virtue of cleanliness. We're taught slogans like Cluttered desk, Cluttered mind. We feel pangs of anxiety when our garage is too dirty. We dust. We fret that our life is too jumbled, so maybe we try a time management system that involves books, software, and iPhone apps. We use these tools for a few weeks, then we fall off the wagon, so we feel more anxiety, then we try them again—this time for *real*—and then they fail again, and then again, until we say, *screw it.* Then we try them again.

But what if, at the age of seven, we were totally right? What if obsessing over cleanliness and order, for some of us, is just a big fat waste of time? This is the argument of Eric Abrahamson, a professor at the Columbia Business School and the coauthor of *A Perfect Mess: The Hidden Benefits of Disorder.* His theory: when someone praises the merits of order, they rarely take into account the *cost* of that cleanup. Desks don't clean themselves. Filing systems take work. (Cleanliness, just like booze, has a trade-off.)

"There are often significant cost savings to be had by tolerating a certain level of messiness and disorder," Abrahamson writes in *A Perfect Mess*. "It's not just that the advantages of being neat and organized are typically outweighed by the costs. As it turns out, the very advantages themselves are often illusionary." If you spend twenty hours cleaning up your desk, he asks us, are you going to get twenty hours back of greater efficiency? (In fact, according to his research, people with orderly desks spend 36 percent more time finding things.) And this obsession for order could have a real psychological downside; his studies found that two-thirds of people report feeling guilty about their messiness.

A Perfect Mess begins with a quote from Einstein, who asks us, "If a cluttered desk is a sign of a cluttered mind, of what, then, is an empty desk?" Let's push the idea further. So maybe your desk is buried under stacks of magazines, books, and empty cups of yogurt. Good news. That shit show is making you more creative. (Maybe.) Here's the theory: the disjointed chaos of a mess could subconsciously nudge your brain away from convention. Where less advanced minds see a moldy slice of pizza, you see "a trigger for nonlinear thinking."

There's evidence to back this up. Kathleen Vohs, a professor of marketing at the University of Minnesota, had a hunch that clutter could inspire our creative juices. She enlisted forty-eight volunteers and then instructed half of them to go into a clean workspace and half of them into a messy one. Then she conducted a brainstorming experiment. She told them to imagine that a ping-pong ball factory, for whatever reason, needed to invent some new uses for ping-pong balls. The volunteers had to write down as many ideas as they could. She also had a set of independent judges score their answers for creativity.

The results? "We found that the subjects in both types of rooms came up with about the same number of ideas, which meant they put about the same effort into the task," explains Vohs in an op-ed. "Nonetheless, the messy room subjects were more creative, as we expected. Not only were their ideas 28 percent more creative on average, but when we analyzed the ideas that judges scored as 'highly creative,' we found a remarkable boost from being in the messy room—these subjects came up with almost five times the number of highly creative responses as did their tidy-room counterparts." Messy has merit.

Procrastination

I'll get to this later.

Napping

We treat sleep as if it's a failure in willpower. The very words "sleeping in," "napping," and "sleepyhead" connote laziness, a lack of purpose, the slob on the couch. We say bad-ass things like "I'll sleep when I'm dead." We make fun of people who go to bed early. In the pre-electricity age of the nineteenth century, the average American slept for 8.5 hours. It's now around 6.5.

"The average person is an hour to an hour and a half sleep-deprived," says Dr. Richard Stack, medical director of the Mercy Sleep Center. He tells me that a full half the population suffers from insufficient sleep, and for working mothers, it's likely as high as 70 to 80 percent. We're on red alert for the obesity epidemic, but we're losing a silent war to the sleeping epidemic.

This has consequences. Research has shown that sleep deprivation—even when it's mild—can erode our cognitive skills, blunt our reaction times, and hamper our memory. It crashes cars. It's linked to obesity; it tricks our metabolism and makes us more likely to overeat. A University of Colorado study found that when people slept only five hours a night for a week, they gained 2 pounds. Or take this quirky little experiment from Sweden: researchers analyzed the way that men shopped for groceries, finding that when the men hadn't slept well, they tended to buy food with higher calories.

It kills our brain cells. A study from the University of Pennsylvania found that when we short-change ourselves on sleep, the damage to our brains could be *permanent*. For mice, at least, sleep deprivation led to a staggering 25 percent long-term loss in neurons. "We've always assumed full recovery of cognition following short- and long-term sleep loss," said Dr. Sigrid Veasey. "Some of the research in humans has shown that attention span and several other aspects of cognition may not normalize even with three days of recovery sleep, raising the question of lasting injury in the brain."

Are you sleep-deprived? Before you answer, consider another study from Penn, this one even more unsettling. The researchers asked volunteers to sleep for only six hours a night for two weeks. No biggie, right? The scientists then asked the volunteers how they felt. The volunteers said, for the most part, that they could function normally. But the data told a different story. The scientists also tested their reaction times and cognitive abilities, finding something startling: the volunteers *performed like people who hadn't slept in two days.* Two takeaways here: (1) A consistent, moderate sleep deficit can be just as bad as pulling all-nighters.

(2) We can be sleep-deprived without realizing it. The doctors concluded that sleep deprivation can, in a cruel twist, fool our brains into thinking we're not sleep-deprived. It's like the drunk guy who insists he's totally sober.

There are, logically, only three ways to crack this problem:

1. Go to bed earlier.
2. Sleep in later.
3. Take naps.

As for going to bed earlier: good for you if you can do it. Please e-mail me and tell me how it's done.

As for sleeping in later: the CDC whipped up an experiment in eight different high schools. They switched the start time from 7:20 a.m. to 8:50 a.m., then monitored the results of these combined eight thousand students. To the surprise of no sixteen-year-old, with the later start time, the students had measurably higher test scores, attendance, and morale—and 70 percent fewer car crashes.

As for napping: it works. Just ask NASA. In the 1990s, NASA performed a study on its pilots, allowing them to take 26-minute catnaps during flight. The nappers showed an improved performance of 34 percent and a stunning 100 percent lift in physiological alertness. Other studies have shown similar results. Napping boosts our physical and mental game. (We benefit most from 20- to 30-minute catnaps—*or* a complete REM cycle of 90 minutes—but not between 30 minutes and 90 minutes, as that would yank us out midcycle and leave us groggy.)

Corporate America is starting to get it. Google installed "sleeping pods" in its offices; the Huffington Post did the same thing.

Others will surely follow. I, too, own a "sleeping pod": I call it a couch. And now it's time to use it.

Fidgeting

I'm a fidgeter. I can't keep still. I'm always bobbing a knee, tapping a foot, or rapping my knuckles against a desk. I've assumed this made me a weirdo, but research suggests that fidgeting can improve our fitness and, bizarrely, lengthen our lives.

"Fidgeting 'Could Prolong Your Life,'" the UK's *Telegraph* announced with cheer. The evidence? Well . . . here it gets a little shaky. Before clicking, I had imagined some meticulous study that plots the life span of fidgeters versus non-fidgeters, concluding that my fellow fidgeters lived to the age of 106 and were 37 percent more likely to marry Keira Knightley. Not quite. But I was thrilled to learn about the Fidget Project, an "interactive art installation touring the UK . . . focusing on the science of sedentary behavior." Launched by Michael Pinsky, a modern artist, the group traveled around Britain and encouraged people to do things like wiggle their bodies and hula-hoop.

Pinsky's manifesto:

> We live in boxes called houses, we move in boxes called cars, we work in boxes called offices, whilst all the time we are looking at boxes called TVs, or perhaps now iPads, PlayStations and smartphones. We move our bodies less and less and if we are not careful we may just fade away. How many times were you told to stop fidgeting when in that box called school?

We need to fidget to survive—let us welcome the Fidgeting Revolution.

Plenty of science backs this up. It's well documented that we live a more sedentary lifestyle than prior generations, and *even if we exercise*, we're still sitting down for a dangerous stretch of time. Our butts love chairs. "Sitting all day long is literally killing us," said the Mayo Clinic's obesity expert, Dr. James Levine, in 2013. "It is bad whether you are morbidly obese or marathon-runner thin. It appears that what is critical and maybe even more important than going to the gym, is breaking up that sitting time."

Studies have shown a direct link between number of hours sitting and likelihood of disabilities, heart disease, diabetes, and lung and colon cancer. A Canadian study at Queens University in Kingston, Ontario, strapped a group of volunteers with accelerometers that measured their steps and movements, then measured their "VO2 max"—the maximum amount of oxygen you can suck in during exercise—as a proxy for cardiorespiratory fitness. They found that the fidgeters—the ones who tended to pace and putter in their daily lives, just going about their business—had the highest VO2 max. They were in better shape. "It's encouraging to know that if we just increase our incidental activity slightly—a little bit more work around the house, or walking down the hall to speak with a coworker as opposed to sending an e-mail—we can really benefit our health in the long term," said the study's lead researcher, Ashlee McGuire. "Best of all, these activities don't take up a lot of time, they're not difficult to do, and you don't have to go to a gym."

Other studies have estimated that fidgeting can burn roughly

300 calories per day—this swings wildly from person to person, of course—which is comparable to a three-mile jog. (Caveat: the word "fidgeting" might be used a little loosely, as there's a difference between rapping your knuckles on a desk and pacing back and forth in a room.) This helps explain the surging popularity of step-trackers like the FitBit, Jawbone, and even the Apple Watch. All of these itty-bitty steps add up.

Complaining

Complaining is stamped in our DNA. It's how we communicate, it's how we solve problems, it's how we rally others to our cause. When you were a baby, you complained to get burped or have your diaper changed. The United States, in a sense, grew from the soil of complaints. To paraphrase our founding fathers: "That King George, he's such a prick about taxation without representation, right? #MeetUpInPhilly."

If we never complain we bottle things up, feed the belly of our resentment, let the wound fester. Psychologist Dr. Robin Kowalski, perhaps the leading authority on the subject, traces the roots of her work to Dr. James Pennebaker, who studied the disclosure of traumatic events. He found that when Holocaust survivors never spoke about the trauma, it compromised their health. "You can see the connection to complaining," Kowalski tells me. "Of course I'm not saying that complaining about the weather is on the same plane as the Holocaust, but the underlying logic is the same. There's cathartic benefit to complaining."

The *type* of complaint matters a great deal. Psychologists split the world of complaints into two different buckets: instrumental and expressive. Instrumental complaining is done with a desire to actually fix a problem. Expressive complaining is just venting, blowing off steam. "When someone's really, really angry with their spouse, sometimes the only person that hears about it is the bartender," says Dr. Guy Winch, author of *The Squeaky Wheel: Complaining the Right Way to Get Results, Improve Your Relationships, and Enhance Self-Esteem*. He suggests that 95 percent of the time, we complain to people who aren't the source of the problem. We can do better.

In one of Kowalski's studies, for example, the researchers asked three panels of people to think about a person they were unhappy with. Then they were asked to write about this wretched person. Each panel was given a different directive for the letter:

Panel 1: Write *to the researchers* about why you're mad at the person.
Panel 2: Write as if you're actually sending a letter *to the person* you're mad at.
Panel 3: Write about what you did yesterday.

The people in Panel 2—who wrote the direct complaints—tested highest in overall happiness. *And they didn't even send the letter.*

I know I'm guilty of too much expressive complaining, not enough instrumental. Take the cable company. I hate Time Warner Cable with the fire of a thousand suns, and I speak with their customer service more than I do my own parents. I later grumble to friends, family, coworkers, or the person unlucky enough to be sitting next to me on the subway. Is this doing any good?

"There can be attention-seeking dynamics that go on. Misery

loves a posse," says Dr. Michael Cunningham, professor of psychology at the University of Louisville. "You may be implicitly seeking a group of people who are willing to join your posse against Time Warner." But this can grow tiring. Is my stream of negativity antagonizing my friends? Am I being *that guy?* Cunningham has a theory called the "allergy of the repetition": when something irritates us, the more we're exposed to that irritant, the more annoying it gets. (That grating Christmas carol might be annoying the first time you hear it, but by the thirty-seventh time, instead of getting "used to it," we're driven to madness.) This is the danger of too much expressive complaining.

Instrumental complaining, on the other hand, is something we should do more of. In *The Squeaky Wheel*, Wench outlines how the customer service industry—a relatively new phenomenon—is powered by complaints. Businesses need them. "A restaurant might have a problematic line cook, or some systemic problem with the food," says Wench. "And because we're uncomfortable with complaining, they wouldn't know it." Complaining about our undercooked steak isn't obnoxious; it's helping them.

COMPLAINING ON SOCIAL MEDIA

A common criticism of the Internet: it's nothing but negativity and cynicism. So, is complaining on social media a good or bad thing?

"It's a positive," says Winch. "You can get validation with it; when you start a hashtag, you're getting emotional validation and you can reach others who feel the same way." (In moderation. This can quickly get annoying.)

And on a more pragmatic level, Twitter has made it easier

to actually address your complaint to the right place. "Twitter has changed the psychological mind-set. If you get bumped from your flight, before you had to e-mail or write a letter. Now you can tweet directly to the airline, and many of them will respond right away."

So let's stop complaining about complaints. (Or maybe do more of it.)

Gossip

Your coworker leans in. Whispers to you. "Did you hear about Graham, from Marketing? Dude was drunk before lunch." You both laugh. Oh, Graham.

There's a reason you like to gossip. And maybe you shouldn't apologize for it. About two-thirds of all conversation is gossip, according to psychologist Robin Dunbar, who traces the roots of gossip to the earliest Homo sapiens. In his book *Grooming, Gossip, and the Evolution of Language*, he suggests that gossip, far from being just a cheap thrill, is the very reason language developed. Just as apes and monkeys used grooming—stroking their fur, petting each other, picking their nits—to build friendships and bond with others, we humans, once we grew in numbers, needed a way to do the same thing. Enter gossip.

Gossip serves a dual purpose in society: it tells us what behavior is permissible; it's a looming threat that keeps all of us in line. In the office, gossip is a more powerful force than any pamphlet from Human Resources. We might not read the fine print on page 42, but we know that if we make out with the hot intern, people will talk. "Gossip reinforces the values of the community,"

Dr. Cunningham tells me. It cues you in to the social norms. "It's a way of saying, 'You can go out and drink, but don't get as drunk as a Kardashian.' It tells you the community's limits."

It's how we learn who we can trust, who's a bad tipper, who's a cheater, who's a slacker. (*If* the gossip is true. Which is always the dark side of gossip.) Recent research suggests that gossip can even impact the state of our emotions. Dr. Robb Willer, a psychologist from Stanford, conducted an experiment. A group of fifty-one "observers" watched other volunteers play a game. Each observer was hooked up to sensors that measured his or her heart rate. Multiple rounds of the game were played. It's possible to cheat at this game, and when the observers witnessed the cheating, their heart rates shot up.

Then the gossip kicks in. Between rounds of the game, the observers, if they chose, could warn future contestants about the cheaters. Some did. And when they did so, their heart rates went down. Takeaway: the gossip had a benefit to their physical well-being. In later rounds of the game, the observers even *paid money* to warn someone about the cheater.

"Groups that allow their members to gossip sustain cooperation and deter selfishness better than those that don't," said Matthew Feinberg, a coauthor of the study. "And groups do even better if they can gossip and ostracize untrustworthy members. While both of these behaviors can be misused, our findings suggest that they also serve very important functions for groups and society." (Gossip, in this sense, is a distant cousin of complaining.)

Game-theory studies have shown that when people are aware of the consequences of gossip, they're more likely to behave honestly. A culture *without* gossip could be less effective. "Imagine a workplace," said Willer, "where an employee's performance could only be seen by individuals in the immediate setting, and those individuals could not pass on what they had seen to other coworkers or supervisors. It would be hard to deter workers from cutting corners ethically or freeloading, working only when they were directly supervised."

All of this refers to what Willer calls "pro-social" gossip. Plenty of gossip is just nasty. For that uglier strain, it's best to listen to one of the earliest writings on gossip, the book of Leviticus, which tells us, "Thou shalt not go up and down as a tale-bearer among thy people."

Laziness

I looked for studies showing that laziness is good for us. I didn't find any in the first two minutes, so I gave up and said, fuck it.

Procrastination

Frank Partnoy is a corporate legal scholar. When researching the origins of the financial crisis, he discovered a story about the top executives of Lehman Brothers who, during the 2005 frenzy of the subprime market, went to an off-site retreat. They listened to speeches from psychology experts, decision making theorists, business school academics, and luminaries like Malcolm Gladwell, who had just written *Blink*.

"Whatever these executives learned was the worst possible thing they could have taken away," Dr. Partnoy tells me. "They went back to their offices and made the worst snap decisions in the history of the financial markets."

This got him thinking: instead of "blinking," could there have been more value in *delay*? Maybe we're thinking too fast, reacting too quickly, and rushing ourselves into shoddy decisions. This led him to research the upside of procrastination. He interviewed hundreds of leaders in business, science, and the military, and this research eventually spawned his book *Wait: The Art and Science of Delay*.

"We're told that procrastination is bad. That when you're putting something off, you should just get it done," says Partnoy, who speaks in a slow, deliberate, almost mesmerizing cadence. I hang on his every word. "But often when you're procrastinating, you're doing it for a good reason. If you never procrastinate, you'll just be an animal responding to instant stimulus."

As a thought experiment, Partnoy asks us to pretend that we're lawyers and we have a brief that's due in thirty days. You could start working on it right now. But you know that it's really only going to take two days to knock it out, maybe four. Partnoy's advice? Put the bastard off as long as you possibly can, because one of the following things might happen in the next thirty days:

- Sometimes the case will get settled anyway.
- Sometimes new data will become available that you wouldn't have had originally.
- And the real benefit, something that happens far more frequently—sometimes a new idea will occur to you.

"We all do our best work in the shower or while sleeping," he says. If you never procrastinate, you never give yourself the downtime to unlock these deeper insights. "In most situations we should take more time than we do," he tells me. "The longer we can wait, the better." It also makes you work more efficiently: why work four hours when you can do it in two? Partnoy's favorite procrastinators range from Pericles to Jon Stewart to Jimmy Connors. "The Greeks and Romans regarded procrastination as something the wise elders did. The leaders of our society are people who sit back and take as much time as possible." There's something to this. In any organization, the lowest rung on the ladder is for the *now! now! now!* burger flippers. As you get more senior you can lounge in the board room, sip brandy, and take as much time as you like to reply to e-mails. You're no longer on the clock—you *are* the clock.

"We're hardwired to react very quickly to information and stimulation," says Partnoy. "Reacting instantly might have been a good hardwired trait when we were out on the Serengeti a hundred thousand years ago, but it often leads us to wrong snap decisions today."

Consider a tennis player. The professional tennis player typically has 500 milliseconds to return a serve. Partnoy argues that what separates the good from the great is not being fast, but *being slow*. Studies of elite athletes show that they wait until the last possible second to pounce on the ball, and this micro-pocket of time gives them an extra opportunity to assimilate new data—the spin of the ball, the wind, its velocity, the opponent's court position. Delays have value.

Just ask a comedian. "When you're trying to tell a joke, there's an optimal amount of delay," says Partnoy, slowing his speech even further. When Jon Stewart is doing a bit, sometimes he'll wait as long as 20 seconds before uncorking the zinger. At this point, it's fair to ask if that really counts as *procrastination*, or is this just the mastering of timing? Partnoy sees the principles as the same. We need to embrace the value of delay, not feel guilty about it. "The optimal delay is not infinite for all decisions—the delay might just be an hour. If you get an e-mail from someone, rather than just respond right away according to instinct, take the time to consider."

There are two flavors of procrastination: active and passive. Active procrastination is the lawyer's conscious decision to delay the briefing; passive procrastination, as you would guess, is the loafing that gets us in trouble—putting off taxes until April 15 (I've done this); going five years without seeing the dentist (also this); or waiting until December 23 to begin Christmas shopping (yep, this too). "I'm not advocating that people just don't do anything, that they lie around on their sofa all day," says Partnoy.

Bummer. I have yet to find a study that finds "lying around the sofa all day" is good for you. But I'll keep looking for one. Tomorrow.

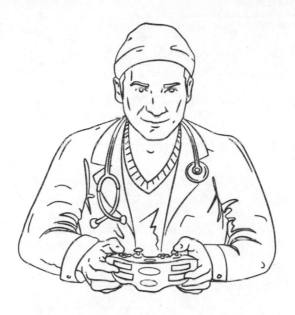

VICE AND DIVERSIONS

Let's think about the phrase "guilty pleasure." What does it even mean? If it's pleasurable, why should we feel guilty? It'd be one thing if our action inflicts harm upon someone else, in which case, yes, we should feel guilty. (Example of an actual guilty pleasure: teenage shoplifting. Theft should bring guilt.) But what about the harmless stuff like TV, video games, pot, web surfing, or even watching a bit of porn? And just how bad is nicotine, really? We'll ask the experts.

Nicotine

Don't start smoking. If you do smoke, quit. Billions of studies have clearly, repeatedly, conclusively proved that smoking leads to things like cancer, heart failure, arthritis, and bad breath when kissing. The CDC says that one in every five deaths is caused by cigarettes. So don't start.

But! While cigarettes are emphatically bad, there are, it turns out, some sneaky health benefits to nicotine.

Dr. Maryka Quik is a neuroscientist. She's the director of the Neurodegenerative Diseases Program at SRI International's Center for Health Sciences, and her research has shown that nicotine, bizarrely, can trigger certain receptors in the brain—neurotransmitters called acetylcholine—which can lower the risk of Parkinson's disease, Tourette's syndrome, and schizophrenia. "The delivery system of cigarettes is very bad. It contains numerous chemical compounds that are toxic. This is what coats the inside of your lungs and makes them blacken in time," she tells me. "But the nicotine alone. . . . If you were to administer the nicotine by itself, that could, potentially, benefit the nervous system. Why do people smoke in the first place? It makes you feel better."

This isn't just theoretical. The data is promising enough that the Michael J. Fox Foundation for Parkinson's Research is funding a study that uses the nicotine patch. "Looking collectively across many studies, it's estimated that current smokers are 60 percent less likely to get Parkinson's than those who have never smoked," says the foundation's website. "Which begs the question: Could there be a drug for PD hidden somewhere within the rolling papers?" As you read the pages in this book, there are 160 patients with Parkinson's wearing either a nicotine patch or a placebo, hoping this might bring them closer to a cure.

A study at Vanderbilt University gives more reason for optimism. In a group of seventy-six people with mild cognitive impairment (elderly who showed signs that they might eventually have Alzheimer's), about half wore a nicotine patch for six months and the others wore a placebo. Then they took tests. The ones with the patch showed improvement in "cognitive measures of attention, memory, and mental processing." But the dosage matters—too much nicotine, just like too much of anything, can backfire. "If you're already functioning fine, but slip down the hill, nicotine will push you back up toward the top," said lead researcher Dr. Paul Newhouse. "A little bit of the drug makes poor performers better. Too much, and it makes them worse again, so there's a range. The key issue is to find the sweet spot where it helps."

Another goofy paradox: while cigarettes are obviously addictive, the nicotine itself might not be. "Nicotine in a cigarette is addictive. But if you take nicotine by a pill, or in a patch, the addictive nature seems to be much, much less, if it exists at all," says Quik. This partly explains why the nicotine patch, for many, fails to help them quit smoking—by definition it's not addictive.

So does this mean that all of us will get a little smarter if we wear a patch? And does smoking actually help the average brain? Not so fast. "In animal studies, nicotine has been shown to increase the growth factors in the brain and, by doing that, it can slow the degeneration caused by a neurological disease," says

Quik. The key phrase here is *slow the degeneration*. There's less evidence (if any) that by releasing dopamine, nicotine helps a normally functioning brain. "We're basically not that certain yet," she says.

"So I shouldn't go out and buy a patch?" I ask her.

She laughs. "Let me put it to you this way. I go to a neuroscientist convention every year, and none of us are wearing nicotine patches."

Pot

This could be a moot point. At the rate things are changing, by the time this book goes to press, pot will be legal in all fifty states, it will be prescribed by doctors as a cure for the common cold, and members of Congress will give televised speeches while openly smoking joints.

But the issue isn't so clear-cut. Not all doctors are game. A 2014 survey from WebMD, which polled 1,544 doctors, found that while the *majority* give pot a thumbs-up, the results are far from unanimous. From WebMD:

- 69 percent [of doctors] say it can help with certain treatments and conditions.
- 67 percent say it should be a medical option for patients.
- 56 percent support making it legal nationwide.
- 50 percent of doctors in states where it is not legal say it should be legal in their states.
- 52 percent of doctors in states considering new laws say it should be legal in their states.

On the one hand, it's worth underscoring that, for some conditions, pot *really does* have a medicinal upside. That's not just a joke. Real studies—by real doctors!—have shown that pot can help treat things like seizures, arthritis, multiple sclerosis, glaucoma, inflammation, and freshman year of college.

But here's the catch: What if it actually changes the wiring of our brains? Or, more troubling, what if it changes the wiring of *teenagers'* brains, in ways that might cause long-term damage? This was the implication of a 2014 study by Dr. Jodi Gilman of Harvard Medical School. Gilman's team used MRIs to study the brains of people who said they smoked a joint at least once a week, and compared them to a control group of abstainers. They were surprised by the results. The pot smokers had differences in the size, shape, and gray matter in two key regions of the brain—the nucleus accumbens and the amygdala—which are linked to emotion and motivation. (The old cliché that pot makes us lazy? It could have some basis in neuroscience.) They also found that the more frequently someone puffed, the greater the changes to the brain.

The study triggered some scary headlines like "This is your brain on drugs," so I tracked down Dr. Gilman to get her perspective. "This is a small study and more research is clearly needed, but currently, we don't know how much marijuana, if any, is safe," she tells me. "This study indicates that there are observable differences in brain structure with marijuana, even in recreational young-adult users. We should be cautious about marijuana and discourage use in adolescents, whose developing brains may be even more susceptible to cannabis-induced changes."

What a buzzkill. But what about all those medical benefits? "I believe that marijuana may have medicinal properties for very specific diseases," says Gilman. "But all medications have side effects, and FDA-approved drugs have been carefully dosed and are required to report all side effects publicly. This has not been done for medical marijuana. Marijuana may very well have therapeutic effects but, just like any other drug, it's probably not safe for everyone. It will be very important for the medical community to weigh the costs and benefits of recommending medical marijuana to patients, especially if they have a family history of psychosis or addiction."

And this brings us to the crux of the Great Pot Debate: is it addictive? As former Surgeon General Jocelyn Elders once said, "Marijuana is not addictive, not physically addictive anyway." That's the catch: *physically addictive.* In the broader context of psychological addiction, well, that's a different story. "Anyone can get addicted to marijuana; there is strong evidence that the earlier people start using marijuana, the more likely they are to become addicted," says Gilman. "Nine percent of users become addicted to marijuana; and when people start smoking as adolescents, this number can increase to about 17 percent. Daily users have a much greater chance of becoming addicted. Also, people report physical as well as psychological withdrawal effects—sleep disruption, headaches, appetite changes, and either weight loss or weight gain, and mood swings." Not something to take lightly. (Then again, for perspective, as *Slate*'s Brian Palmer reminds us, "That's low compared with dependence rates for other drugs: More than 15 percent of people who drink become alcoholics, and 32 percent of people who try cigarettes get hooked.")

So, yes, pot might be addictive and it might change our brains, but alcohol, too, is addictive and might change our brains. It's naive to think that pot is the Great Devil, but it might be equally naive to call it harmless. "There are strong opinions on both sides of the marijuana debate, which is understandable," says Gilman. "However, whether people are pro- or anti-legalization, they should not be anti-science."

Video Games

According to my female friends, there's nothing less sexy than a grown man playing video games. "It's a deal breaker," one friend told me. "It's almost as bad as being a racist."

But according to new research, video games have a 79 percent chance of making men more attractive, and are proven to help them last 47 percent longer in bed. Okay, that's a lie. But it's true that in recent years, study after study has shown that video games—in moderation—can stretch our brains and confer sneaky benefits. They're more than just a guilty pleasure. The issue isn't black and white. As the neuroscientist Dr. Daphne Bavelier told the BBC, "We know there are good sugars and bad sugars, and we don't discuss whether food in general is good or bad for us. We need to be far more nuanced when we talk about the effects of video games."

So for anyone looking to justify your addiction to Madden, here's a bit of fodder:

1. *They make us think.*

When I was a kid, I enjoyed the simple pleasure of mashing buttons to get Mario past the dragon. It was mindless. But today's games? They're complex, challenging, and they even test our creativity. There's a reason that Minecraft sold 7.9 bajillion copies of the *guidebook*, let alone the game itself. Video games are puzzles, and puzzles help us learn. Back in the day, when you played Tecmo

Super Bowl, you just lobbed the ball to Jerry Rice and padded your stats. Today's Madden is hard: elaborate playbooks, detailed blocking schemes, infinite ways to run your offense. It's more chess than checkers. In a study from UC San Francisco, researchers had older adults, ages sixty to eighty-five, play a game, called NeuroRacer, where they drove virtual 3-D cars through obstacles. The scientists hooked the volunteers' brains to EEGs, had them play for one month, and then found improvements in their memory, attention span, and ability to multitask. Bonus? Some of this improved performance lasted *six months after* they played the game.

2. *They're associated with good behavior in kids.*

In 2014, researchers from Oxford surveyed five thousand kids, quizzing them as to how often they played video games. They found that when kids played for an hour or less each day, they tended to have greater empathy and, in general, were better behaved than kids who never played. They were happier. "There's a wide range of reasons to think that some level of exposure to electronic games might be advantageous to young people," lead researcher Andrew Przybylski said. The catch is the predictable one: when kids played games for more than three hours, they tended to have problems with attention span, they were less satisfied with life, and they were 5,000 percent more likely to get stuffed in lockers.*

3. *They can help get kids in shape.*

A 2014 experiment from the University of Queensland in Australia found that when obese kids were given an "active" gaming system, like the Wii, after a four-month weight management

---

*Correlation versus causation alert. This just shows an "association." It could be that well-adjusted kids tend to gravitate toward video games in moderation. As far as epidemiological studies go, this one's pretty loosey-goosey.

program, they lost twice as much weight as a control group. "If your child is in a weight management program and using an active gaming system, your child is more likely to get more active during that program," explained the Cleveland Clinic's Dr. Sara Lappé. "The active gaming system can help your child to get up and moving and get the heart rate up." Is it healthier for the kids to actually go out in the sunshine and play soccer? Probably. But some kids, for whatever reason, just aren't into sports. An active video game can dupe them into burning calories.

4. *They're good for our eyes.*

One study found that playing Tetris helps people with amblyopia, otherwise known as lazy eye. Other research has shown that video games—particularly action games—could boost our eyes' ability to detect contrast. "Action gamers may have stronger vision. They can better distinguish between different shades of grey, called contrast sensitivity, which is important when driving at night and in other poor visibility situations. . . . They also have better visual acuity, which is what opticians measure when they ask you to read lines of ever smaller letters from a chart at a distance," writes Nic Fleming in BBC.com's "Why Video Games May Be Good for You."

5. *They make good doctors.*

A study from the University of Rome found that when doctors played Wii, they tended to become better surgeons. For a month-long experiment, one group of doctors played games like Wii Tennis and Ping-Pong, and one group of doctors just acted like normal adults. Then they tested their technical and motor skills. As the authors of the study conclude, "The Nintendo Wii might be a helpful, inexpensive and entertaining part of the training of young laparoscopists, in addition to a standard surgical education based on simulators and the operating room." So the next time you're choosing a doctor, ask for her top score on Wii Bowling.

And on and on. It's a long list. Various studies have demonstrated that they can improve reaction times, spatial relationships, motor skills. They might provide pain relief. They reduce stress and depression. They help kids with illnesses like autism and Parkinson's disease. It's fair to say that with each passing year, more research emerges to show that video games—especially the ones that are complex, challenging, or physically active—do more than just kill time and repel women.

So, guys, the next time you're playing *Grand Theft Auto*, if your girlfriend walks in on you just as your character is, for example, in a virtual strip club with a naked stripper, who's grinding on your virtual crotch, just tell your girlfriend with a straight face, "Video games are a puzzle, and puzzles help us learn."

Web Surfing

Videos of kittens make you more productive. This is according to *science*. Such was the discovery of Dr. Don J. Q. Chen, a researcher from the National University of Singapore, who found that when office workers took breaks to screw around online, they were actually more productive, more engaged, and made fewer errors.

Here's some of the evidence: Chen asked a group of students to do some mundane work for twenty minutes (reading papers and highlighting the letter E, which is more intellectually stimulating than some office jobs I've had), and then split them into three groups:

Group 1 kept working for ten minutes.

Group 2 did whatever they wanted (except for web surfing) for ten minutes.

Group 3 surfed the web for ten minutes.

Then all of them got back to work and highlighted more E's. The web surfers were the fastest and they made the fewest mistakes.

This seems almost too good to be true. I reached out to Dr. Chen for his thoughts and he told me, "Web surfing is a form of micro break. It is a positive distraction that allows individuals to temporarily take their minds off work demands and work stress. When individuals switch from doing something that is stressful and demanding (such as work) to something that is fun and pleasurable (like web surfing), they experience increases in positive affect (emotions). Positive affect is related to improvements in mental acuity."

Not all web breaks are created equal. Whereas web surfing was linked with a boost of productivity, *personal e-mail* was not. One is fun, the other's a chore. "E-mailing imposes additional demands on employees' cognitive workload since they need to spend attention on drafting e-mail messages," says Chen. This taps into why web surfing isn't simply a micro break; it might be a uniquely beneficial form of micro break.

Let's not overlook the obvious: Web surfing is easy. It's passive. We just click and scroll and zone out. It's easier to skim celebrity gossip than it is to force ourselves to give a shit about our coworker's broken stove. "A web-surfing break is more effective in managing stress than talking to colleagues or taking a water cooler break," Chen tells me. "Individuals in our study generally regarded web surfing as being more pleasurable than chitchatting with others. An extension of this finding would be that the more pleasurable

one finds an activity, the more effective that activity is in helping one manage stress."

So what's the optimal amount of time we should waste online?
Dr. Chen's research suggests that ten minutes is "sufficient to make
a difference to productivity." And eight hours should be sufficient
to get you fired.*

Porn

How is porn good for you? Well, no one's saying it's going to help
cure cancer. It's not going to make you live longer. And it's not a
surefire way to save your marriage. If you're busted watching porn,
I don't recommend saying, *"Honey, I'm watching this orgy for us,
I'm doing this to SAVE OUR FAMILY!"*

So why is it in the book? Because porn is demonized. It comes
with shame, guilt, and embarrassment. Porn has been accused of
ruining sex lives, poisoning marriages, desensitizing men, objecti-
fying women, inciting sexual violence, creating unrealistic expectations of what a woman's body should look like, and causing "porn
addiction."

All of this is rubbish, says Dr. David Ley, a psychologist and
author of *The Myth of Sex Addiction.* "Can porn be dangerous? The
only negative effects of porn are on people already disposed toward
violence. In them, it may increase the chance of sexual violence.

---

* So how to square this with the idea that multitasking can be bad for you? This
sounds like a classic health paradox. But the two might be compatible. Instead
of darting back and forth between work and the web, focus on one thing—and
only one thing—for a sustained period of time, then switch.

In others, it has no effect," he tells me. "In fact, in multiple international studies, access to porn leads to a decrease in sex crimes, including rape, sexual abuse, and exhibitionism."

To further research the topic, I thought about watching three hours of porn every day for a year, but since that would be anecdotal, we'll make do with a 2007 study in Croatia, where a survey of 650 men found that porn viewers had the same level of sexual fulfillment, relationship satisfaction, and emotional intimacy as porn abstainers. (That same study, however, did find that viewers of *violent* porn tended to experience less emotional intimacy—so skip the snuff films.) "If anything, there is an inverse causal relationship between an increase in pornography and sex crimes," writes Dr. Milton Diamond in a 2009 study. "Objections to erotic materials are often made on the basis of supposed actual, social or moral harm to women. No such cause and effect has been demonstrated with any negative consequence." (I remain a little skeptical.)

One charge against porn is that it leads to depression. Another is that if men watch it too much, they become numb to real women, as they're lost to the fantasy world of 32DD. "Some people do experience negative effects when they increase porn use to cope with loss, loneliness, stress, etc.," says Ley. "But research shows that porn comes *after* negative life events and depression, *not* before, as is often speculated by the sex addiction crowd. This means increased porn use is not a cause but an effect. This is very important." (Yet another example of correlation versus causation.)

As for any negative consequences to porn addiction? This affects less than 1 percent of men and women, according to Ley's study, which happens to include my favorite line of any technical research paper: "More [pornography] viewing has been related to greater likelihood of anal and oral sex and a greater variety of sexual behaviors. This increased breadth of sexual behaviors could arise by increasing a person's feeling of empowerment to suggest new sexual behaviors or by normalizing the behaviors."

There's also an argument to be made that porn is a vehicle for diversity. (Try using this argument next time you're caught watching *My Big Fat Greek Bedding*.) The index of PornHub.com, for example, includes Latina, Indian, Japanese, Squirt, Handjob, Gay, Mature, Interracial, and Creampie. Anyway that's what a *friend* told me. "Porn increases awareness and acceptance of a range of sexual differences, orientations, and desires," says Ley. "The common belief that porn is all 'pneumatic blond Barbies' is debunked. Porn includes a tremendous variety of body types and appearances, and can be quite affirming."

Okay, and fine, while we're on the subject, we might as well address . . .

Masturbation

No joke. Studies have linked masturbation and/or frequent orgasms to a lower risk of prostate cancer for men, lower risk of endometriosis for women, and lower risk of heart disease for everyone. It might even help prevent cervical infections and type 2 diabetes. It also tends to feel good.

I reached out to Dr. Gloria Brame, author of *Sex and the Self*, who has written extensively on the health benefits of self-pleasure. "People who know how to give themselves orgasms are usually better lovers as adults, in part because they feel more comfortable with nakedness and know what gives them pleasure—especially important for women: in my experience, the women who struggle the most with orgasm when they're with lovers are uptight about masturbation, too. It has a myriad of benefits emotionally and psychologically, because it is nature's own stress buster."

How common is it? As Michael Castleman writes in *Psychology Today*, "An old joke observes that 98 percent of people masturbate—and the other 2 percent are lying," That might not be far from the mark. It's by no means a rigorous study, but a British company called Gossard (a maker of lingerie) surveyed one thousand women between the ages of eighteen and thirty, finding that *92 percent* of them partake. "Women now have the confidence to prioritize their personal needs both socially and in the workplace," said a spokeswoman. "Our survey results demonstrate how women's sexual behavior has evolved in relation to this new role and environment."

In her role as a therapist, when a patient has issues, Brame asks for their "sex history," which is basically a "chronology of sexual behaviors from childhood through today. The deeper the problems, the deeper those questions go." And it starts with masturbation. "I start by asking people when they first started masturbating, whether they still do, and how they feel about it," she says. "Those questions help me understand not just how they feel about masturbation but their overall 'state of libido' and their feelings about their own genitals and about sex. People who are very masturbation-negative usually have the most difficulty with a fully pleasurable sex life."

TV

What's better for you, books or television?

Of course this question is preposterous; books give us Shakespeare; television gives us *The Biggest Loser.*

But then let's ask a different question: If you have six hours of leisure time, are you better off reading *The Da Vinci Code* or watching *The Wire*?

"Popular culture has, on average, grown more complex and intellectually challenging over the last thirty years," writes Steven Johnson in a book that's naturally near and dear to my heart, *Everything Bad Is Good for You,* which focuses on the sneaky upsides of television, video games, and the Internet. "Where most commenters assume a race to the bottom and a dumbing down—'an increasingly infantilized society,' in George Will's words—I see a progressive story: mass culture growing more sophisticated, demanding more cognitive engagement with each passing year."

Watching *The Wire* isn't mindless. Following the story takes work—it forces the brain to fire the neurons. Historically, TV was a distinctly "passive" viewing experience, and Johnson argues that even with the classic shows—he cites *Murphy Brown, Frasier,* and *The Mary Tyler Moore Show*—"the intelligence arrives fully formed in the words and actions of the characters onscreen." We're not asked to fill in the gaps. Sam Malone cracks a joke; we laugh.

Our current shows are different. Ambiguity abounds. Our brains are shaken from their sofas and forced to figure things out. Jokes are more layered. They take patience. "The social network of *24* mirrors the social network you frequently encounter in the small-town or estate novels of Jane Austen or George Eliot," argues

Johnson, who wrote this in 2005, before *24* went downhill. (Swap in *Orange Is the New Black* or *True Detective* and it still works.) "The dialogue and description are more nuanced in those classic works, of course, but in terms of the social relationships you need to follow to make sense of the narrative, *24* holds its own." Clarification: I'm not making the case that TV should replace books. It shouldn't. But historically, just like wine and chocolate, television is viewed as a "guilty pleasure," when maybe we shouldn't feel that guilty.

Okay, so maybe the higher-end TV is good for our brains, but what about the crap? Some studies suggest that even the junk has merit. "Perhaps people turn to television not to 'zone out' or escape, as is often believed, but to replenish resources lost doing exhausting activities," explains researcher Jaye L. Derrick, whose team found that when volunteers even *thought* about their favorite TV shows, they had higher levels of self-control or willpower. Prior research has shown that willpower, at times, is a finite resource. It can be depleted. One study showed that when people had to fight their urge to eat a cookie, afterward they had less willpower to complete a series of tests and puzzles. "Self-control is like a muscle," Derrick tells me. "When people have exerted self-control to do something effortful, they become temporarily fatigued and are less able to exert self-control on subsequent effortful tasks." This new research suggests that watching TV has the opposite effect of refusing the cookie: when people thought about their favorite TV shows while completing a logic game, they were better able to complete a second round of puzzles. Derrick concludes that "media use can have unexpected psychological benefits. Television, movies, and books can be more than mere leisure activities; in some cases, they fulfill needs, like restoring self-control, that people are reluctant or unable to fulfill through other means."

But who am I kidding? We all know TV isn't that bad. Let's look at something more controversial.

Ecstasy

Meet David Nutt. He's a British scientist. A leader in the field of neuropsychopharmacology (the study of how drugs impact the brain), Dr. Nutt was a high-ranking member of the UK government, serving as chair of the Advisory Council on the Misuse of Drugs. (He's kind of a big deal.)

He raised some eyebrows when he wrote an essay titled "Is Ecstasy More Dangerous Than Horseback Riding?" recommending that the government downgrade ecstasy from a class A drug (such as heroin, cocaine, PCP) to class B (like pot), concluding that "drug harm can be equal to harms in other parts of life. There is not much difference between horse-riding and ecstasy."

Let's look at the math. We can assess the damage of ecstasy versus horseback riding across a few different metrics:

Metrics: Death Rates

By his estimate, "a rider can expect a serious accident once in every 350 hours riding." Horseback riding causes about ten deaths per year, and ecstasy causes between ten and fifty, depending on who you ask.

So far: ecstasy is more dangerous.

Metric: Overall Physical Damage

Ecstasy causes 2,000 hospital admissions each year. Horse racing: 5,700 serious accidents.

Edge: Horse racing is more dangerous.

Metric: Absolute Risk

When you tally up the other factors (injury to others, psychological damage), he finds the total number of "adverse effects" to be 6,000 in both categories. "Ecstasy pills, however, are far more common than riding, with police estimating that about 60 million tablets are taken per year," he writes in his book *Drugs Without the Hot Air*. "Six thousand out of 60 million means that ecstasy causes roughly one case of acute harm every 10,000 episodes: every 10,000th pill, someone is likely to get hurt." How is that relevant? The odds of hurting yourself with an ecstasy pill are only 1 in 10,000 . . . but 1 in 350 for riding a horse.

Let's be clear: He's not saying we should hit the clubs and wave our glow sticks and go do Molly, or whatever it is the kids are calling it now. But he's trying to untwine the *absolute risk* from the perception of risk. He's closing the Perception Gap. "Ecstasy is a harmful drug—in no way should this chapter be interpreted as saying anything different," he clarifies. "But how harmful? As harmful as drinking 5 pints of beer? As harmful as getting on a motorbike?"

He's a natural provocateur. In 2007, he led a study that ranked the Top 20 Most Harmful Drugs. When measured by the harm *to the user*, the usual suspects topped the list: heroin, crack, meth. Then they ranked the drugs a little differently. The scientists also captured the harm to others—including car accidents, violence, abuse—and perched at the very top of the list, higher than pot, ecstasy, cocaine, or even heroin . . . came alcohol.

Parliament was not pleased.

In 2009, he was sacked.

But what about the impact of ecstasy on the brain? Isn't it addictive? Doesn't it cause memory loss? Not according to a 2011 study from Harvard. This research, led by Professor John H. Halpern, argued that prior studies—which suggested that ecstasy damaged the brain—were polluted by unfair comparisons of test versus control groups. The old studies found that ecstasy users were less healthy than ecstasy abstainers, but it just so happened that ecstasy users were the rave kids who were also getting drunk and taking other drugs. There were too many confounding variables. So for the 2011 Harvard study, the researchers did three things different: They . . .

- Excluded people who were heavy users of other drugs or alcohol.
- Required that "all participants be members of the 'rave' subculture."
- Tested all participants "with breath, urine, and hair samples at the time of evaluation to exclude possible surreptitious substance use."

The goal was to strip away the confounding variables, so only ecstasy use would explain the differences. The conclusion? No brain damage. "Essentially we compared one group of people who danced and raved and took ecstasy with a similar group of individuals who danced and raved but who did not take ecstasy," said

Dr. Halpern at the time. "When we did that, we found that there was no difference in their cognitive abilities."

This result was unsettling for many. But not for a certain expert in neuropsychopharmacology, who, upon learning of the results, said, "I always assumed that, when properly designed studies were carried out, we would find ecstasy does not cause brain damage."

(The British government remains unimpressed: at the time of this writing, he remains sacked.)

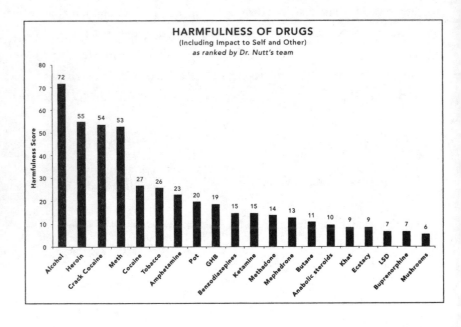

HARMFULNESS OF DRUGS
(Including Impact to Self and Other)
as ranked by Dr. Nutt's team

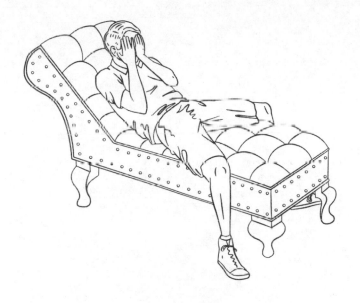

BAD
MIND-SETS

We kick ourselves for being stressed out, feeling down, worrying too much, failing, or getting angry. In the same way that we carve the grocery store into Good Foods and Bad Foods, we chunk our brains into Good Emotions and Bad Emotions. We've seen that food isn't so black and white. Neither is our psyche. This has its upsides. . . .

Stress

Why does stress get such a bad rap? I mean besides the fact that it can cause heart attacks, hives, insomnia, impotence, and diarrhea?

Stress is necessary. It keeps us alive. It makes us function. "Scholars in science and philosophy, for centuries, have known that stress causes physical illness. But stress is also a mechanism by which we cope with society," says Dr. Robert London, a psychiatrist who specializes in stress-related disorders. When your body detects something stressful—like, say, a bear running toward you—the brain shoots a quick message to the pituitary gland, and this, in turn, unleashes your cortisol hormones. Cortisol gets shit done. It's basically a steroid that temporarily makes you stronger, faster, sharper, and more likely to outrun a bear. Fight or flight.

"Short-term stress can make you more efficient in the moment," London tells me. "Let's say someone's coming to visit your home or apartment, and you're stressed about cleaning it up. That's good stress—it helps you speed up, and maybe remember things you haven't put away." This can make us more productive.

The problem, of course, is when the stress is chronic. We can't make a habit out of running from bears. "The problem in modern times is that our body's stress response is regularly triggered even though our lives are not in danger," says London. So it's no surprise that according to the CDC, 90 percent of all illnesses are related to stress.

Anyone who has played video games will be familiar with the Turbo button that only lasts for a few seconds; if you mash Turbo all game, your Energy Bar will shrink. For a more dignified analogy, the president of the American Institute of Stress, Dr. Paul J. Rosch, compares stress to the tension in a violin string. "Not enough produces a dull, raspy noise and too much results in an annoying shrill or snaps the string. However, just the right amount of stress creates pleasing sounds."

Most of this has been known for some time. Recently, though, scientists are exploring whether the way that we *think* about stress can flip it into a positive. It's all in the way you frame it. "Can changing how you think about stress make you healthier? Here the science says yes," says Dr. Kelly McGonigal, psychologist and author of *The Upside of Stress,* in a 2013 TED talk. "Your heart might be pounding, you may be breathing faster . . . but what if you viewed them as signs that your body was energized and it's preparing you to meet this challenge?"

Her theory is backed by multiple studies, like an experiment at the University of Wisconsin, where researchers asked twenty-nine thousand people two questions: (1) How much stress do you have? (2) How do you think stress impacts your health? Then they studied the mortality rates of this group over the next eight years. They found that when people had a high level of stress *and* they believed that stress negatively impacted their health, their mortality rates were 41 percent higher. But when people had a high amount of stress but *didn't believe* it negatively impacted their health, that higher risk of death vanished. A 2012 study from Harvard reached a similar conclusion.

	HIGH STRESS	LOW STRESS
Think stress is bad	Unhealthy	Healthy
Think stress is good	Healthy	Healthy

"The harmful effects of stress on health are not inevitable," concludes McGonigal. "How you think and how you act can transform your experience of stress. When you choose to view your stress response as helpful, you create the biology of courage."

Translation? The very fact that you read this essay—and might view stress more positively—might actually boost your health.

Introversion

What do Abraham Lincoln, Bill Gates, Rosa Parks, and Gandhi have in common?

All of them were introverts.

Many of us are. At least one in three Americans are introverts, even if we're forced to hide our true selves, grit our teeth during cocktail parties, and conform to a world that's rigged for the outgoing. People use the word "introvert" as if it's a personality defect. Introverts are made to feel inadequate. If we'd rather curl up with a book instead of going to a birthday party, then there must be something wrong with us.

"Introversion—along with its cousins sensitivity, seriousness, and shyness—is now a second-class personality trait, somewhere between a disappointment and a pathology," writes Susan Cain in *Quiet: The Power of Introverts in a World That Can't Stop Talking*. "Introverts living under the Extrovert Ideal are like women in a man's world, discounted because of a trait that goes to the core of who they are. Extroversion is an enormously appealing personality style, but we've turned it into an oppressive standard to which most of us feel we must conform."*

Which is a shame. As Cain demonstrates, research has shown that when we meet people who are outgoing and talkative, our natural bias is to assume they're smarter. But that bias is flawed. One study, for example, asked a group of college students to solve math problems as a team. After the math-fest, each student was asked to rate their teammates' intelligence. "The students who spoke first and most often were consistently given the highest ratings, even though their suggestions (and math SAT scores) were no better than those of the less talkative students," observes Cain. This means that good ideas get lost in the noise of extroverts.

In another introvert manifesto, *Quiet Influence*, Jennifer Kahnweiler makes the case that globalization, flattened organizations, and the rise of digital media creates a land that's ripe for the introverted Wozniaks of the world. "Introverts, as particularly thoughtful users of social media, may be well ahead of the game," suggests Kahnweiler. "They have been drawn to social media because it lets them use their strength and better manage their communication." (You don't have to be an extrovert to go viral, unless you're making a sex tape.) Kahnweiler says that introverts have the four P's that can make them effective leaders:

---

*What if you're not sure if you're an extrovert or introvert? Then we're in the same boat. Whenever I've taken introvert-extrovert personality quizzes I split my answers right down the middle—I crave my alone time, but I also talk too much at dinner parties, which, technically, makes me what the experts call an ambivert.

Introverts prepare.

Introverts are present.

Introverts push themselves.

Introverts practice.

Selfishness

New research suggests that selfishness can make us happy . . . but only if we're *forced* to be selfish. This removes the stigma. Researchers from Penn conducted this cute little experiment: they gave two hundred people an envelope and split them into three groups:

Group 1: Told they were given $3. (Whoo hooo!)

Group 2: Told they were given $3, but they had to donate it to the UN Children's Fund.

Group 3: Told they were given $3, and they can *choose* whether to pocket the money or donate it to the Children's Fund.

Afterward, the group was given a survey to assess their mood. The happiest group? The ones who were given the $3 cash, then *forced to keep it*. They were measurably happier than the ones who were given $3, but had the choice to give it to charity. "The study shows that when you force someone to do something selfish, they actually like it," researcher Jonathan Berman tells me. "But if they choose to act selfishly, they feel bad about it. What this suggests is that people often *want* to act selfishly, but avoid doing so because they don't want to feel selfish. Or to put it another way, people often prefer selfish rewards, but don't want to feel selfish in the process."

Besides, is it really so bad to be selfish? "If you completely neglect what's in your own interest, you're not going to be in a position to help others," says Dr. Barry Schwartz, psychologist and author of *The Paradox of Choice.* "You need to be healthy, energetic, and well-educated in whatever domain you choose. All of that involves cultivating the self. A doctor who neglects himself and gets burnout can't help any patients." There's a reason that flight attendants tell us that in the event of an emergency, we should first use the oxygen masks on ourselves, and only then, after we're okay, help our children. This doesn't mean we want our kids to die. It just means that altruism, for all its merits, is useless if we're dead.

Disgust

What is it, exactly, that brings humanity together? Is it our capacity to love, our shared ancestry, or the coding of our DNA?

It might be our revulsion of poop.

In her book *Don't Look, Don't Touch, Don't Eat: The Science Behind Revulsion,* Dr. Valerie Curtis makes the case that at a very primal level, it's our disgust that keeps us clean, guides us to avoid parasites, and even informs our code of ethics. Without disgust we are beasts.

Humans are probably "the only species to be able to imagine ourselves being disgusted in the future," explains Curtis. "This has huge evolutionary benefits—we can stay home when there's plague about to avoid encountering sick people. We can choose to put food in the refrigerator today because we can imagine a rotten mess tomorrow."

This isn't just theoretical. If you are reading this book, chances are you're in a first-world country, have access to soap and water, and have showered at least once in the past month. But when I spoke with Curtis, she told me about her work in Africa and India, in poor villages, where hygiene is so bad that it leads to sickness and death. Two-thirds of all deaths in Africa are caused by infections. So she worked with a PR agency on a "disgust campaign" to gross people out, showcasing a dirty man who puts worms in his food and has diarrhea. If the villagers are disgusted by this, hopefully, they will wash their hands and stay healthier. Disgust can be a force for change.

Disgust helped us evolve. "Our distant ancestors who tended to avoid feces, nasal mucus, and bad-smelling food did better on average in the reproduction lottery; they were healthier, mated more often, brought up more children to sexual maturity, and hence had more grandchildren," explains Curtis. "And these grandchildren, the descendants of the disgusted, were more disgustable themselves—and so on, till the present day, and us."

Nearly all humans, across nearly all cultures, are disgusted by the same things. All of us cringe at body odor, rotten chicken, the Jonas Brothers. Curtis's research found that we also tend to share a "metaphysical disgust" that "affects our attitudes toward cloning and to [genetically modified] foods, our judicial systems, our politics; and that it even affects our product-buying behavior." But this isn't always a positive. A culture's disgust of "abnormal sex," for example, might have sprung from a desire to avoid sexually transmitted diseases, but now this can spawn homophobia. Disgust, like everything, has trade-offs.

Failure

Just as we beat ourselves up when we eat "bad food" like choco-late or red meat, we tend to beat ourselves up when we fail. It's the same dynamic. And just as there's an upside to chocolate and red meat, there's an upside to failure.

We need failure. It sharpens us. Inspires us. Brings out the best in us. Yes, maybe that's something of a cliché, but it's one of those clichés that has the ring of truth. "Failure is feedback. Just like the serrated edges of the side of the road can help you from nod-ding off, failure can be a wake-up call," Dr. Jeffrey Rubin tells me. Too much is problematic (see: Chicago Cubs), but a moderate amount is necessary. If you're never failing, you're not taking enough risks.

Failure is the backbone of the scientific method. We cook up a hypothesis, we test it, and if our experiment fails, we challenge that hypothesis and make it better. Or, if you want to play with seman-tics, you can take comfort in the old Thomas Edison quote, "I have not failed. I've just found 10,000 ways that won't work."

Taking a more philosophical stance, failure is what defines us. "Ultimately, our capacity to fail makes us what we are; our being essentially failing creatures lies at the root of any aspiration. Fail-ure, fear of it and learning how to avoid it in the future are all part of a process through which the shape and destiny of human-ity are decided," writes Dr. Costica Bradatan, a professor of philo-sophy, in a *New York Times* op-ed. "We are designed to fail."

Worrying

It's natural to worry at the airport. You worry about the security line, you worry about checking luggage, you worry about delays.

But not me. I don't care if the FAA recommends we get there ninety minutes early—*please;* twenty minutes is plenty. On the rare occasions when I reach the gate with more than seven minutes to spare, I turn around, wander through the terminal, flip through magazines, and maybe get my shoes polished. I'm the last person to board the plane.

Ninety-five percent of the time this serves me well. But sometimes, in that niggling 5 percent, I'll miss my flight. This is profoundly stupid. When I was 35 years old—no longer a naive college kid—I had to call my mom and give her the news.

"Hi, Mom. I won't be there tonight. I missed my flight."

"Oh," she said, hiding her disappointment. "It's no big deal, sweetie. What happened?"

I wanted to tell her that there was some car accident. Or that Delta screwed me over. Or that we had some terrorist threat. Instead, the truth was simple: I just didn't worry enough.

And according to certain studies of the brain, this might even mean that I have a lower IQ. In 2012, scientists from SUNY Downstate Medical Center measured the brain activity in two groups of people—one group was a control, and one group had general anxiety disorder. They monitored the metabolism of something called choline in the brain's white matter, which is an indication of brain activity. Their takeaway? Worrying is linked with higher intelligence.

"While excessive worry is generally seen as a negative trait and high intelligence as a positive one, worry may cause our species to avoid dangerous situations, regardless of how remote a possibility they may be," explained the lead researcher, Dr. Jeremy Coplan. "In essence, worry may make people 'take no chances,' and such people may have higher survival rates. Thus, like intelligence, worry may confer a benefit upon the species."

That squares with a 2013 study from the University of Sussex, which found a link between worrying and the brain's "systematic processing," suggesting that when we worry, we are more likely to trigger the left front lobe—the chunk of the brain that's associated with analysis. In this model of neuroscience, there are two different ways of thinking: *heuristic processing*, which is an intuitive, gut-level decision; and *systematic processing*, which is more deliberate.

Translation? Worriers tend to be more thoughtful. We're more likely to trigger heuristic processing (gut decisions) when we are confident in our actions, and this overconfidence can get us in trouble. "Systematic processing is more likely to be deployed when individuals feel that they have not reached a satisfactory level of confidence in their judgment," writes Dr. Suzanne Dash, "and this is similar to the worrier's striving to feel adequately prepared, to have considered every possible negative outcome/detect all potential danger, and to be sure that they will successfully cope with perceived future problems." This might be why other studies suggest a link between worrying and longer life spans.

Worrying makes us think. As psychiatrist Dr. Cunningham tells me, "Worrying is a form of problem-solving. You are mentally going over an issue and looking for a form of leverage, control, or anticipation." And like everything, of course, worrying needs to come in moderation.* Too much makes us panic for no reason; too little makes our ideas undercooked.

Spite

Say hello to the Spitefulness Scale. Created by Dr. David Marcus of Washington State University, it's the world's first attempt to measure our level of spite. It's built from a questionnaire that asks whether you identify with certain petty scenarios. My favorites:

- "If my coworkers were going to get larger raises than me, then I would prefer it if none of us received raises."
- "I would be willing to take a punch if it meant that someone I did not like would receive two punches."
- "If I am going to my car in a crowded parking lot and it appears that another driver wants my parking space, then I will make sure to take my time pulling out of the parking space."
- "It is sometimes worth a little suffering on my part to see others receive the punishment they deserve."

It's this last statement—helping others get their comeuppance—where spite reveals its magic. "Spite may have an adaptive function, in terms of basically keeping other people honest," Marcus

---

* It's time to create a drinking game. Every time you see "in moderation," you should drink. Because drinking is healthy for you. In moderation.

tells me. "It can be a way to make sure that if there are other individuals acting inequitably, they might be more at risk." Spite can keep others in line. (It's similar to the gossip dynamic.) That's backed by some game theory research from Tufts University, which found that *just a bit of spite* helped the overall equity of a computer-simulated economy.

Spite might even have something to do with our sex lives. Tim Wadsworth, from the University of Colorado, analyzed the survey results of fifteen thousand people and explored the correlation between happiness and the response to "How often do you have sex?" In results that will shock no one, people are happier when they get more nookie. Then it gets more interesting. He also found that we tend to be happier *if we think we're having more sex than our friends.* "Having more sex makes us happy, but thinking that we are having more sex than other people makes us even happier," he explains.

So imagine two different scenarios:

1. You have sex twice a week, but your friends are having sex four times a week.
2. You have sex once a week, but your friends are only having sex once a month.

Wadsworth's results suggest we'd be happier with number two. Spite is sexy.

That said, while spite might serve a useful function for society as a whole, it does not, generally, benefit you personally. Marcus's study found that "Spitefulness was positively associated with aggression, psychopathy, Machiavellianism, narcissism, and guilt-free shame, and negatively correlated with self-esteem, guilt-proneness, agreeableness, and conscientiousness." Who's more likely to be spiteful? "Men reported higher levels of spitefulness than women" and "younger people were more spiteful than older people."

What about the idea that spite can be a healthy outlet, somehow purging you of bad mojo? Marcus isn't so sure. "I'm skeptical of the 'catharsis hypothesis,' because when we do lash out and hurt others, we rarely feel better about ourselves," he says. "In the long run, I doubt that it leads people to feeling happier."

One last thing. Of course I had to take this spite test myself. How could I not? Marcus sent me the questionnaire and some instructions—cautioning that because I've already spoken to him about the overall issue, my results might be a tad biased—and I answered the seventeen questions. I was disappointed to score a 64. Did that mean I failed? I e-mailed him my score, and he replied, "This would be at the ninety-ninth percentile across our combined samples, which is pretty spiteful." Ninety-ninth percentile, baby! Finally I found something I could win. Pleased with myself, I sent the test to the next most spiteful friend I know . . . who scored a 65. He just barely beat me, and this made me spiteful.

Anger

Researchers from Berkeley took a group of 175 people and asked them to do a little role-playing: one game was confrontational, one was collaborative. Before the start of the role-playing, the volunteers were induced to feel either angry (by listening to death-metal music or recalling angry memories) or happy (by listening to peaceful music or recalling serene memories), and some had a neutral emotion. Each volunteer was allowed to choose if they wanted to be happy or angry.

The results? When it came to confrontation, in the long term, the volunteers who *chose to be angry* experienced a rosier sense of well-being. "Emotions can help us pursue our goals. Emotions were likely designed to help us adapt more efficiently to changing environmental circumstances, and given this, emotions serve important functions for us still," says Brett Ford, a coleader of the research. "For example, anger promotes aggressiveness and asser-tiveness, and can help people confront others more successfully. So, if I have a goal to confront someone, it might actually better serve that confrontation goal for me to feel angry in that moment— compared to, say, happiness, which promotes collaboration and friendliness, and may actually backfire in this context."

They also found that people who are *chronically* angry, how-ever, experienced a lower overall sense of well-being. It should be used in short bursts. Targeted. "Anger is not a very socially appro-priate emotion . . . and yet it can still be useful," Ford tells me. "People who (a) know it's useful, (b) know the contexts for which it's useful, and (c) are willing to want to feel it in those contexts . . . are more likely to have higher well-being."

The usual caveats apply. Too much anger (just like too much talking about caveats) is counterproductive. "Anyone can become angry—that is easy," says Aristotle. "But to be angry with the right person, to the right degree, at the right time, for the right purpose, and in the right way—this is not easy." Or to quote a researcher from the Dagobah system, Dr. Yoda: "Anger leads to hate. Hate leads to suffering. Suffering leads to the dark side."

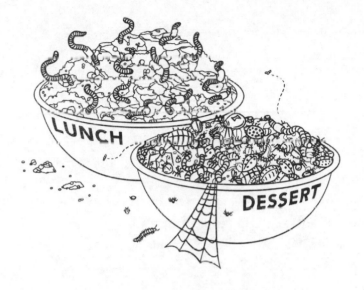

(ALMOST) EVERYTHING ELSE

Here's one of the strangest things in the book: it's true that "obesity" is linked with a million health problems, but once someone has been diagnosed with diabetes, weirdly, if they're obese, they tend to *live longer*. That's one of the many paradoxes we'll zip through in this section—fevers can help us, dirt can protect us, pesticides can save us, even bugs can feed us.

Obesity

Obesity is a problem. A serious one. Some quick facts:

- Over 70 percent of Americans are overweight.
- Over 35 percent are obese.
- 70 percent of all heart disease can be linked to obesity.
- Half of all adults with type 2 diabetes are obese.

None of this is controversial. The experts all agree. So make no mistake: the message of this entry is not *You should get obese!*

And yet . . .

About a decade ago, Dr. Carl Lavie, a star cardiologist who has authored over eight hundred medical publications, spotted some trends in mortality rates that were rather, well, funky. In short: it's true that if you are obese, you have a higher risk of being diagnosed with something like diabetes. But here's the twist. Being *diagnosed* with a disease is not the same thing as *dying* from it, and once people are diagnosed with a cardiovascular disease, the odds flip-flop, and the obese are less likely to die from it.

In other words, you're more likely to be diagnosed with diabetes if you're obese, but out of that filtered population (people diagnosed with diabetes), the fat people tend to live longer. Enter the obesity paradox. "Over the past decade a multitude of highly respected studies from around the globe have confirmed the obesity paradox, and the reluctant scientific community has been forced to rethink its definitions of fat—and consider how it could actually have positive attributes under certain circumstances," Lavie writes in his wondrously contrarian book, *The Obesity Paradox*.

The obesity paradox can be seen in patients with arthritis, cancer, diabetes, and AIDS. It's baffling. Being fat is awful for our health in every way until, all of a sudden—boom!—it has the power to save our lives.

One explanation: some types of fat are protective. "The fat that clutches your vital organs—what we call visceral fat—is not the same as the fat we attribute to thunder thighs, cellulite, and big butts," explains Lavie. The obese have plenty of this protective visceral fat (think of it as the styrofoam inside a box, protecting a fragile lamp), while the skinny catwalk models lack this essential cushion. It's a deep-rooted cultural problem. We fetishize skinny. We covet being *thin* when we really should be focusing on being *fit*. "Fat is not the devil," Lavie tells me. "We can no longer say what people and many doctors have said for long times—that thinner is necessarily healthier. Fitness is more important than fatness for long-term health outcomes."

As most of us know all too well, it can be damn near impossible to lose fat around our hips and thighs. And that's probably a good thing. "The fat that accumulates around women's hips, thighs, and buttocks . . . are excellent retainers, sucking up extra energy and storing it ardently, thereby protecting the liver," explains Lavie. "So while we may despise saddlebags and thunder thighs, take heart; they might be good for you."

The crux of the obesity paradox, according to Lavie, can be explained by the fact that "fit versus unfit" matters more than "fat versus thin." It's possible to be considered "obese," which is technically defined as a body mass index north of 35, and still be in decent cardiovascular shape. Exercise matters. You know how it seems that sometimes, even if we're jogging three or four times a week, we still can't melt away the pounds? That effort isn't wasted. It still strengthens the heart. "Some individuals may try to manage their weight and health through diet alone, shunning fitness, and they experience metabolic consequences similar to if they were morbidly obese," he explains. "People can be obese but metabolically healthy and fit, with no greater risk of developing or dying from cardiovascular disease or cancer than normal-weight people."

He's not urging people to get fat. But the pendulum has swung too far and now we demonize fat, dread it, use it as a scapegoat. It's the wrong conversation. Lavie concludes, "It's much better for your health if you're fat and fit than thin and unfit." This echoes a sentiment from the mid-1990s; to quote noted scientist Sir Mix-a-Lot, "I like BIG BUTTS, and I cannot lie! Baby! Got! Back!"

Dirt

Dr. Sera Young, an anthropologist, traveled to a tiny island off the coast of Zanzibar, East Africa, to interview pregnant women about their eating habits. While sitting in a sunny outdoor kitchen, she asked a pregnant woman what she liked to eat.

"Every day, twice a day, I take a chunk of earth from this wall and, well, I eat it."

Wait, what?

She asked the pregnant lady if she had heard her correctly. Dirt? Yep. Dirt. Young was intrigued. Immediately she changed the focus of her research, spending the entire summer interviewing people in this small island. Many of them ate dirt. This craving is called pica.

The pregnant lady gave her a new mission in life, which resulted in the world's most comprehensive study of geophagy, the practice of eating dirt. This culminated in her book *Craving Earth: Understanding Pica—the Urge to Eat Clay, Starch, Ice, and Chalk.*

"Eating dirt has been reported on every inhabited continent and in almost every country," Young tells me. Her database now has 480 distinct instances of cultures eating dirt. We see it in kids, we see it in grown-ups, and we see it in the writings of Hippocrates, two thousand years ago.

So what's the appeal? Her team had two initial hypotheses: (1) The hunger hypothesis. This was quickly ruled out, as the dirt-eating cultures had plenty of normal food. (2) The nutrition hypothesis. This, too, was ruled out, as the dirt lacked nutritional benefits like iron or zinc.

The likely winning answer: protection. Maybe the dirt protects our gut, lining our stomach and serving as a buffer, of sorts, from parasites. This is why the practice is more common with pregnant women. "You would typically want food to cross into your bloodstream, but in early pregnancy, you are particularly susceptible to things like tannins," says Young. (Tannins are, technically, plant-based polyphenolic molecules that are often found in things like tea and red wine.) The dirt binds with the mucus lining of the gut, serving as an extra line of defense from potentially dangerous substances.

This doesn't mean that dirt is always healthy. (Again, trade-offs.) First off, these properties only apply to "clean dirt" (the soft, clay-like, spongey dirt that's rich and earthy), not the contaminated stuff that many of us see in cities. "Some people are addicted to dirt, and even talk about it like it's a drug," she says "They'll say, 'I've been clean for several weeks, and then I went to a friend's house . . .' There are a number of dangers, and they're not trivial."

In the grander scheme of things, it's not *that* much of a stretch to reason that, okay, if certain cultures eat clumps of dirt like skittles, maybe we shouldn't be so paranoid about getting our food a little dirty? Maybe we're going overboard in our zeal for hand sanitizers? We quickly enter the Hygiene Hypothesis, an entire wing of health that argues that when we never let our kids get dirty, or expose them to bacteria or viruses, they never beef up their immune systems. Young is a believer. "It's important to pay attention to cleanliness. I'm not suggesting not bathing. But we think that we're giving our children a gift by being *so sterile*, and this has a cost. If you go to Bed Bath & Beyond, those apple and cherry pie scented [hand soaps] are so unrecognizable to how we, as humans, have evolved," she says, then laughs. "My children are dirt-bags, and it's fine."

Pesticides

In a rigorous scientific survey, on Facebook, I asked my friends a simple question: "Are you worried about pesticides in food?"

A sampling of the responses:

- "Absolutely. Why would you eat an apple with chemicals if you can eat one without?"
- "YOU should worry. There are some major testicular development risks.

- "No. I probably should care, but I am too busy rolling my eyes when people scold me for not caring."
- "Not for myself, just for the people working on the farms. Though I do always give fruit and veggies a cursory rinse to make myself feel better."

Even though this informal "survey" is biased and lazy, it does illustrate our range of emotions on pesticides. Many of us are not sure what to think, or we're ashamed of our ignorance, or we're convinced that pesticides are dangerous and we pay a premium to avoid them.

This next response seemed to resonate: "I am not worried, only because I feel like I have enough problems to worry about. No scientific data to back up my stance." If we're not alarmed about pesticides, the assumption is that *we're just ignorant*—we haven't read the science—and that if we knew the full story, we'd be terrified.

But what if that's just not the case? What if the science says, basically, the risk is essentially zero? "It seems obvious that genetically engineered, chemically abetted food would be somehow corrupt: less natural, perhaps even dangerous. How could pesticides not cause cancer, right? That's what my gut tells me. The problem is, that isn't what the data tells me," writes Taffy Brodesser-Akner in *Pacific Standard*. "I know there's no *harm* in buying organics, except for the extra cost. Spending that extra dollar protects me from the threat that I'll later regret it, from the fear that the scientists will turn out to be [wrong]."

The key issue: yes, nonorganic fruit contains pesticides. It has chemicals. But as a 2012 meta analysis from Stanford University shows, these levels are so infinitesimally small that they can, according to many, be ignored. The dosage is small. The absolute risk is tiny. As Joseph Schwarcz, director of the Office for Science and Society at McGill University in Montreal, tells NPR, it's a mistake to "equate the presence of a chemical with the presence of risk. . . . Where is the evidence that these trace residues are dangerous?" Another study, this one from UC Davis, concluded the same thing: "Our findings do not indicate that substituting organic forms of the dirty dozen commodities for conventional forms will lead to any measurable consumer health benefit." (The "dirty dozen," of course, refers to produce that has relatively higher level of pesticides. The Environmental Working Group lists them as apples, strawberries, grapes, celery, peaches, spinach, sweet bell peppers, nectarines, cucumbers, cherry tomatoes, snap peas, and potatoes. Plenty of experts, such as Dr. David Katz, still suggest buying organic for the dirty dozen, just in case. As always, there's no consensus.)

Yes, pesticides *in high dosage* could be a threat, but they are, in the end, something that is sprayed for our protection. "Let me be clear about one thing: I'm all for reducing pesticide use. But we can't forget that pesticides are used for a reason, too. We have been reaping the rewards of pesticide use for decades. Higher yields due to less crop destruction. Safer food because of reduced fungal and bacterial contamination. Lower prices as a result of increased supply and longer shelf life. Protection from pests that carry deadly diseases. Invasive species control, saving billions of dollars in damages—and the list goes on," reasons Christie Wilcox in *Scientific American*. "Yes, we need to manage the way we use pesticides, scrutinize the chemicals involved and monitor their effects to ensure safety, and Big Ag (conventional and organic) needs to be kept in check. But without a doubt, our lives have been vastly improved by the chemicals we so quickly villainize."

This isn't letting pesticides off the hook. For the farm workers—who are exposed to a dramatically steeper dosage—the risk could be higher. It's also true, as my friend Annie reminds me, that pesticides pose a real health risk to bees.

Takeaway: if you are a bee, buy organic.

Fevers

"Fever phobia." In 1980, the term was coined by Dr. Barton D. Schmitt, a professor of pediatrics at the University of Colorado, who wrote a study that concluded, "The great concern of parents about fever is not justified. Health education to counteract 'fever phobia' should be a part of routine pediatric care."

Thirty years later and we still have the phobia. According to a survey from *Pediatrics*, 56 percent of parents are "very worried" about the effects of fever, even though, as the American Academy of Pediatrics says, "Fevers are generally harmless. In fact, they can be considered a good sign that your child's immune system is working and the body is trying to heal itself."

It's counterintuitive. I've never been a parent, but I suspect that if my imaginary baby, little Hakeem Olajuwon Wilser, was crying and burning up and looking like he's on death's doorstep, I would have the only appropriate reaction: panic. This would likely be a mistake. "Fever can indeed be scary, and any fever in an infant younger than three months is cause for major concern because of the risk of serious bacterial infections," explains Dr. Perri Klass, a professor of pediatrics at New York University, in an op-ed. "But in general, in older children who do not look very distressed, fever is positive evidence of an active immune system, revved up and helping an array of immunological processes work more effectively."

Certain viruses and bacteria (called "microbes") flourish in the body's normal temperature, so when the body cranks up the heat, it helps burn the microbes away. If you cool the body too quickly, you're playing into the microbes' hands. In 2011, the AAP conducted a sprawling study on fevers and concluded that "there is no evidence that fever itself worsens the course of an illness or that it causes long-term neurologic complications. Thus, the primary goal of treating the febrile child should be to improve the child's overall comfort rather than focus on the normalization of body temperature."

While we're on the subject of illnesses with kids . . .

Allergies

One of my best friends, Cody, has a daughter with a food allergy. It's not a simple one. Her condition is called "T-cell mediated immune response" or "T-cell mediated allergies," which means she's not able to eat soy, dairy, wheat, nuts, most berries, red meat, shellfish, a few different vegetables, and pretty much anything processed using the chemicals and artificial ingredients most people eat every day.*

As Cody tells me, "Her face will break out, there will be blood in her stool or she'll have diarrhea, and she'll be a little crabby for

---

*Score a point for organic food. Maybe *overall* it doesn't make a difference for most people, but there are certainly exceptions. So much of health is case by case.

a few days because all of this causes a not-insignificant amount of pain. That blood will have come from ulcers that will have broken out in her esophagus and stomach as her body reacts to what it perceives as a threat." They've had many trips to the hospital. It's expensive. It's nerve-racking.

According to the CDC, between 4 and 6 percent of all the kids in the United States have a food allergy. (This increased by 18 percent from 1997 and 2007, and no one is quite sure why.) Each year, food allergies send about thirty thousand people to the hospital.

So what, exactly, is the good news?

Traditionally, scientists have thought that allergies are the result of what happens when our immune system gets confused, misfires, and gets activated by a harmless substance, like peanuts. But a leading immunologist at Yale University, Dr. Ruslan Medzhitov, is turning that old model on its head. As he tells me, "The old model is not entirely wrong, but it's definitely incomplete. If you think about every possible symptom of allergic disease—vomiting, coughing, sneezing, runny nose, teary eyes—all of these things have one thing in common: *expelling something out of the body.*"

Our bodies expel things for a reason. If you drink a gallon of spoiled milk, it will cause you to vomit or spend your morning on the toilet. The vomiting itself isn't bad—it's protective. We don't want rotten milk in our bellies.

"Now imagine that you come in contact with poison ivy," Medzhitov continues. "You're itching. And you realize it's because you got stung." So far so good. Here's where it gets interesting. . . .

"Now imagine that you're wearing clothes, and you don't know that there's a chemical on the clothes that's reacting to your skin cells, and it's making you itch. You might think that there's something wrong with you." In other words, even though you can't pinpoint the cause of your itching, your body is acting to protect you. The itching is helpful.

"Okay, so why do we have allergies?" I ask.

"Evolution is concerned with reproductive success, and only that," he says. "Evolution isn't concerned with feeling well, having headaches, or feeling happy. All of that is secondary."

He asks us to imagine that we have two options:

1. We feel very healthy and we feel very happy, but at the same time, we're vulnerable to infections.
2. We have headaches and we feel lousy, but at the same time we're very resistant to infections.

"Evolution would select the latter, and it would eliminate the former."

If you follow this chain of logic, the point is that allergies are somehow protecting us, *even if we don't know the culprit.* It's possible there are toxins, irritants, or some other foreign substances that allergies are warding off. We vomit to expel spoiled milk, we have allergies to protect ourselves from some unknown substance. The fact that we don't know what it is doesn't mean it's not protective.

Others have raised this theory before. Years earlier, a researcher named Margie Profet theorized that allergies exist to protect us and have unknown benefits, suggesting that the "immune response known as 'allergy' evolved as a last line of defense against the extensive array of toxic substances that exist in the environment in the form of secondary plant compounds and venoms." This was largely ignored at the time. "Scientists have generally confirmed an inverse relationship between allergies and many types of cancer, but struggle to explain the observation," writes Mike Martin in *Psychology Today*. "Studies have shown allergies slash ovarian cancer risk by up to 30 percent and leukemia by 40 percent. Cancers of the lung, pancreas, colon, and more than a dozen other areas of the body reflect the same 'inverse allergy' effect."

This might not be of much practical use to my friend Cody and his daughter, and in fact, when I told Cody about this insight, he said, basically, "you're full of shit." Fair. A theoretical benefit sure doesn't feel like much when your daughter is in the hospital. It was a reminder that just because something *might* have some abstract upside, that doesn't mean it's *actually good*, and it can be very, very, very bad. Deadly. This made me imagine the mother of an alcoholic who died in a drunk driving accident, and I thought of this mother reading the breezy essay on bourbon, then bursting into tears. So it's a fine time to reiterate that while this book highlights the wacky, surprising, contrarian findings in health, it does not, therefore, mean that everything bad is good and everything good is bad. Cigarettes still kill. Vegetables still matter.

Okay, for a lighter topic, let's look at how BPAs might cause deformities in infants!

BPAs

BPA stands for Bisphenol A. It's a chemical that's used to make plastic. Cups, cans, Tupperware, even baby bottles. It's feared by many that BPA causes:

- Higher rates of cancer
- Obesity
- Diabetes
- Insulin resistance
- Heart attacks
- Hormone swings
- ADHD
- Brain malfunctions

And as most new parents and soon-to-be parents know, there's concern that BPAs can flummox the development of unborn children.

This is, to use precise medical language, some scary shit. The trillion dollar question, though, is this: *in what dosage?* It's one thing for a study to examine rats and show that, at certain levels, BPAs can turn the rats into pigs. It's something else to show it in humans.

I phoned up risk expert David Ropeik, a professor at Harvard and the author of *How Risky Is It, Really? Why Our Fears Don't Always Match the Facts.* "Because it affects unborn children, BPAs have a sharp emotional resonance," he tells me. But is the concern warranted? "The world's top regulatory bodies have rigorously analyzed all of the science that is well done on BPA and determined that even with the low-dose effects it can have, it doesn't need to be regulated." So what explains the controversy? "But the people who promote the fear of BPA call every one of those science bodies 'corrupt.'" He calls this the Perception Gap: the difference between actual risk and the perception of risk. It's the same gap we've seen with GMOs and pesticides.

Misinformation abounds. Consider the movement for BPA-free baby bottles. In response to pressure from health activists, Walmart yanked the BPA-polluted baby bottles from its inventory, and other retailers soon did the same thing. Health advocates cheered.

A big win, right? We've just made our babies safer! But as Ropeik tells me, the real concern about BPAs was the impact on *the development of the fetus.* "People rang the alarm about BPA, and how does society respond? By saying 'Wow, Oh my god! It's bad for babies! Let's ban BPA from baby bottles!'" he says. "But fetuses don't drink out of bottles. We've eliminated an exposure that has nothing to do with the risk, and *by making ourselves feel safe,* we've failed to eliminate the exposure to Moms." Another irony: A 2015 study from *Environmental Health Perspectives* found that two of the main *replacements* for BPA—Bisphenol S (BPS) and Bisphenol F (BPF)—have the same impact on the body as BPA, suggesting that "BPA Free," essentially, is meaningless.

This is a recurring pattern in the book. (Especially in the flip section—the bad news about what's good for you.) By making ourselves feel good about changing one tiny thing, we're more likely, at times, to miss the big picture. The perception gap causes problems. In his book, Ropeik points out that in the months immediately after 9/11, "a lot of people were so afraid of flying that they drove to distant destinations instead. Driving, because it offers a sense of control, feels safer, but it's a more dangerous way to travel. In the three months following September 11, the death toll on the roads rose significantly compared to what was statistically normal for that period." This caused between three hundred and a thousand additional deaths. Or something more recent: We obsess about Ebola running wild in the United States, but then, at the same time, we fail to get our kids vaccinated.

Less sensational, but the same dynamic: we hear that blue-

berries have an antioxidant that trims the risk of neurodegenerative diseases, so we pat ourselves on the back for tossing this
"superfood" into our bowl of cereal . . . ignoring that this same
bowl of cereal has 45 grams of sugar. The blueberries make us feel
healthy. Driving makes us feel healthy. Choosing bottles that are
BPA-free makes us feel healthy. But we're just misdiagnosing risk.

As Ropeik puts it, the BPAs in plastic are "tiny, tiny, tiny
doses—parts per trillion, more or less." It's so small that, according
to most research, it doesn't move the needle of human health.

The counterargument? Once, not too long ago, the U.S.
government said there was something else that didn't move the
needle of health: cigarettes.

Sun Exposure

I'm not what you'd call a "tanner." I come in only two shades: pasty
white or hot pink. Ethnically, I'm a mix of German, Irish, French,
British, maybe a dash of Czech—a mutt—which makes me the
whitest person on the planet. (One clinical trial that proves my
whiteness: the dance floor.) It's in my blood. My grandfather, for
instance, avoided the beach even though he owned a beach house.
My family keeps Banana Boat in business.

Skin cancer—from mild to deadly—runs in both sides of my
family, and I know it's only a matter of time before I pay the piper.
When I was a teenager, the sun roasted my back so completely that
it blistered, then formed bubbles, then I couldn't sleep, and then,
when I went to work at the grocery store, my boss sent me home.
Not because I asked him to. He sent me home because customers

were complaining about the blood that oozed from my shirt. (Another upside of complaining.)

This is all preamble to say that I'm well aware of the traditional risks of exposure to sunshine, so I was shocked to see headlines like "Sun Exposure Benefits May Outweigh Risks, Say Scientists." Specifically, a British study from the University of Edinburgh suggests that sunlight triggers our body's release of nitric oxide, which lowers blood pressure. And lower blood pressure means a lower chance of strokes. One thing this study has going for it is that it's not just an epidemiological comparison of two populations, but an actual clinical experiment: they took twenty-four volunteers, blasted them with ultra-violet rays from sunlamps, and measured their blood pressure. The blood pressure went down. (Maybe this is why surfers and beach bums are so chill?) "We suspect that the benefits to heart health of sunlight will outweigh the risk of skin cancer," said the lead researcher, Dr. Richard Weller. "The work we have done provides a mechanism that might account for this, and also explains why dietary vitamin D supplements alone will not be able to compensate for lack of sunlight."

Vitamin D, of course, is the other perk of sunshine. (Along with light, energy, and all life on planet Earth.) In Australia, Dr. Rachel Neale followed a group of seven hundred people with high sun exposure, and then followed a comparable group of seven hundred people with low sun exposure—ensuring the groups were of the same age and had the same male-female split—and found that the sunbathers had a 24 percent lower risk of pancreatic cancer. So far so good. But here's the really wonky thing: if you have sun-sensitive skin (like mine), sun-exposure decreases the odds of pancreatic cancer even more—*by 40 percent*.

"The sun is healthy for us in a number of ways. It leads to the production of vitamin D in the skin; vitamin D is important for the maintenance of healthy bones and may also play other roles in our body," Dr. Neale tells me. "The sun also influences our circadian rhythm and our mood. There is some evidence that the sun may affect our immune system with both beneficial and harmful effects."

And there's the rub. *Both beneficial and harmful effects.* How do we know which is which? "We are thus in a difficult position of trying to find a balance between the benefits and harms of sun exposure, and there are many scientists around the world working on this issue," Neale tells me.

Hmmm. Fair. So how long should I be out in the sun?

"The optimal amount of time in the sun will depend on a person's age, skin type, the ambient UVR reaching the Earth's surface, past history of skin cancer, body surface area exposed. Finding a one-size-fits-all message is going to be very difficult."

Ain't that the truth.

Sadness

It's healthy to be sad. This is the message from Dr. Joseph Forgas, a social scientist from the University of New South Wales, who, after conducting experiments for nearly twenty years, has found that sadness can sharpen our memory, improve our thinking, and make us less likely to stereotype.

In his 2013 study, *Don't Worry, Be Sad! On the Cognitive, Motivational, and Interpersonal Benefits of Negative Mood,* Forgas reveals some experiments that suss out the impact of sadness on stereotyping. He asked a group of people to read a one-page philosophical essay, then he split the volunteers into two groups:

1. In some cases, the essay showed a picture of a casually dressed woman as the author of the essay.
2. In some cases, the essay came with a picture of a "tweedy, bespectacled man."

Forgas reasons that "a young unorthodox-looking woman is less likely to be seen as a competent philosopher than a middle-aged man." (Clarification: He's not saying there's any truth to this stereotype, he's merely acknowledging its existence.) Would this (dumb) stereotype influence the results?

It depends on whether they were happy or sad.

Before reading the essay, one group's mood was manipulated to be sad (by asking them to reminisce about sad events), and one group was manipulated to feel happy (by asking them to reminisce about happy events). The happy judges did indeed stereotype, and tended to like the essay better when it showed the tweedy bespectacled man. But the sad judges didn't have this same bias.

His team found the same insight with a far more provocative experiment. Using a computer first-person-shooter game, he instructed people to only shoot at targets who were carrying a gun. Some of the targets were white; some were wearing a turban and appeared Muslim. Sometimes the targets held a gun; sometimes they held a coffee mug. The shooters were more likely to pull the trigger on Muslims carrying coffee mugs than on non-Muslims carrying coffee mugs. (Forgas calls this the "turban effect.") The more interesting takeaway is that when people were in a positive mood, the turban effect was even greater, but when they were feeling negative emotions, this actually *reduced* the stereotype.

What could explain this? It goes back to the framework of the brain that splits our mind into two chunks: 1) The part called heuristic processing that makes gut reactions and snap decisions; and 2) The part called systematic processing that takes its time and uses logic. (We saw this back in the section on Worrying.) System #1 is lazy. It just goes with the flow. And it's even lazier when we're happy. "When in a good mood, people become more intuitive and more creative but also less vigilant and more prone to logical errors," explains Daniel Kahneman* in *Thinking, Fast and Slow*, which explores this two-system model of the brain. "A good mood is a signal that things are generally going well, the environment is safe, and it is all right to let one's guard down. A bad mood indicates that things are not going very well, there may be a threat, and vigilance is required." So to bring this full circle, if we're sad, we're more likely to fire up System #2 and avoid lazy stereotypes.

Takeaway. If someone's a racist, punch them in the mouth so they will be sadder, and therefore less likely to stereotype. (Even if Fargas's theory is flawed, on the upside, at least you've punched a racist in the mouth.)

Bugs

In the summer of 2013, the UN Food and Agriculture Organization unleashed a 200-page report that extolled the benefits of eating insects, suggesting they could be the food of the future.

This is less crazy than it sounds. By the year 2050, the world's population is expected to grow to 9.6 billion (up from roughly

---

*Kahneman won a Nobel Prize and is one of the founding fathers of decision-making theory and behavioral economics. His book is magnificent.

7 billion today), but that will be accompanied by only a 0.000000 percent growth in land. This is a stubborn problem. We need land to do things like grow cattle and raise corn. "For the first time in human history, food production will be limited on a global scale by the availability of land, water and energy," warned Dr. Fred Davies, the senior science adviser for the U.S. Agency for International Development. "Food issues could become as politically destabilizing by 2050 as energy issues are today."

Enter bugs. They're high in protein, they're packed with vitamins, and they're more ecofriendly than a gluten-free kale-enriched organic-wheat-germ non-GMO non-BPA grass-fed free-range smoothie. In other countries there are already 2 billion people eating insects.

I sought guidance from the unofficial king of bugs, Phil Torres, an entomologist and science correspondent for Al Jazeera America. "I think most kids go through a stage of loving to play with bugs. I just never grew out of it," Torres tells me. As a kid he went to butterfly camps during the summer, fell under their spell, and then spent years in the Amazon rain forest, researching insects and identifying new species. He also eats them for dinner.

Torres is a good-looking, charismatic guy who does a ton of TV appearances. (In other words, he doesn't fit your "worm-eater" stereotype.) "In many cultures bugs aren't eaten as a backup food source; they are eaten as a treat or a primary dish," he says. It's estimated that about 1,900 species of insects are consumed around the planet. "There was no 'shaking-off' a bug-eating taboo; they simply have eaten bugs for generations just as many other cultures have eaten chicken or fish." His personal favorite is the fresh cicada. "Sauté them with garlic and you have a legitimately delicious protein source, heartier than mushrooms and healthier than beef."

It's worth spending a moment on the obvious: *bugs are everywhere.* This is important. As Michael Pollan illustrates in *The Omnivore's Dilemma,* everything you buy in the supermarket has a long, looooonnng way to go between the granaries of Iowa and the shelves on aisle 13, and each step of that journey requires another shot of energy. The cows must be fed, the milk must be cooled, the crates must be shipped. The system is vast. But as the Food and Agriculture Organization says, insects have a high "food conversion rate." Crickets, for example, need "six times less feed than cattle, four times less than sheep, and twice less than pigs and broiler chickens to produce the same amount of protein." The FAO therefore sees insects playing three potential roles: consumed directly, like a kid eating worms; consumed indirectly in recomposed foods "with extracted protein from insects"; and consumed by feedstock—bugs could be the food that feeds our food.

"They emit minimal greenhouse gases, they can be raised vertically in towers unlike cows, which need vast grazing areas, and their waste can easily be used as fertilizer," says Torres. "I truly believe insects are the sustainable protein of the future: eat bugs to save the world."

Admit it, this still sounds sort of gross. But as Torres points out, two hundred years ago, there's another food that we found disgusting: lobster. "There were actual laws here in America restricting how many lobsters could be fed to prisoners in a week, as too many was deemed cruel. Lobsters have come a long way; I believe insects are not far behind."

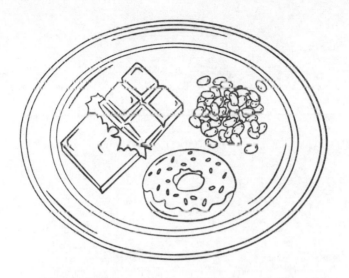

MORE FOOD

Part of the secret of success in life is to eat what you like and let the food fight it out inside.—Mark Twain

Steak

Meet the Inuit. Their very existence has frustrated the health industry for decades. Living in the punishing colds of the Arctic, they eat a diet that's almost entirely meat, fish, and fat. Almost no vegetables. Almost no fruit. Almost no carbohydrates.

A typical day's menu:

Breakfast: Meat.
Lunch: Meat.
Dinner: Meat.

Here's why they're so damned problematic for the world of modern nutrition: the Inuit are healthy. Even though roughly 70 percent of their calories come from fat, observational studies have shown that, relative to us, they tend to have healthier hearts. They live long lives. (Did the words "observational studies" ring some alarm bells and make you think, "Correlation versus causation alert!" *Ex*cellent.)

This paradox has been around for quite some time. In 1906, a man named Vilhjalmur Stefansson, an anthropologist from Harvard, decided to live with the Inuit for a year. He came away impressed. How were they so healthy eating so much fatty meat? The experience stuck in his craw. As Nina Teicholz shares in *The Big Fat Surprise* (seriously, read this book), as an experiment, Stefansson later decided to spend an entire year eating only meat. His contemporaries mocked him. People worried for his health. Now let's think about this for a moment; it's one thing to do a stunt diet like a juice cleanse or a raw-food diet for a week or a month, but this crazy bastard was willing to go an *entire year* without any bread, potatoes, apples, vegetables, bagels, pasta, orange juice, or pancakes. He somehow convinced a buddy to join him. A hospital checked their vitals before the year began. Then they ate meat, more meat, and more meat. Then more meat.

"At the end of a year, both men felt extremely well and were found to be in perfect health. Half a dozen papers published by the scientific oversight committee recorded the fact that scientists could find nothing wrong with them," reports Teicholz. "The men were expected to contract scurvy, at the very least, since cooked meat is not a source of vitamin C. Yet they did not, probably because they ate the whole animal, including the bones, liver, and brain, which are known to contain that vitamin, rather than just the meat. For calcium, they chewed bones, just as the Inuit did."

How is this possible? While it's in vogue to glorify things like avocados as "superfoods," you could make the case that meat is the original superfood. It's loaded with nutritional goodies. "Ever since the 1960s, when it was first argued that animal products could be bad for our health because they contain saturated fat, nutritionists have typically refrained from pointing out that meat contains all the amino acids necessary for life, all the essential fats, and twelve of the thirteen essential vitamins in surprisingly large quantities," writes Gary Taubes, one of the planet's staunchest defenders of meat. "Meat is a particularly concentrated source of vitamins A and E, and the entire complex of B vitamins."

You might ask, yes, okay, so this steak eater survived for one

year, but how did he feel? Did he get sick? He did actually get sick.
Once. This happened after he was encouraged to strip the meat of
its fat. Happily, this illness was "quickly cured by a meal of fat sir-
loin steaks and brains fried in bacon fat," says Teicholz. Also? He
lived until the age of eighty-two.

Eggs

*Eggs are high in cholesterol. Eggs cause heart attacks. Eggs make us
fat.* This is what we've been taught for decades. Eggs, like their red-
meat cousins, have been seen as dangerous, fattening, and something we should consume only in the tiniest of doses, like Reality
TV. We purge yokes. We request egg-white omelets.

But just as we see with red meat, eggs, too, are making a comeback. A 2013 meta-analysis of 263,938 people found that when
people ate an egg every day, their risk of heart attack and strokes
increased by 0.00000000000 percent. The eggs didn't make a
difference.

Not only are eggs just "not bad for you," they're loaded with
the good stuff. "The egg is a powerhouse of disease-fighting nutrients like lutein and zeaxanthin. These carotenoids may reduce
the risk of age-related macular degeneration, the leading cause
of blindness in older adults," writes Dr. Kathleen M. Zelman, a
nutritionist for WebMD. "And brain development and memory
may be enhanced by the choline content of eggs."

I have my own hot-and-cold relationship with eggs. Since college, every morning, I ate the exact same thing for breakfast: cereal. And not the junky cereal like Froot Loops, but the "good
stuff" that you get at Trader Joe's that has less than 3 grams of fat.

I did this for years. And during that entire time, every morning, around 10:30 a.m., my blood sugar plummeted and I needed a midmorning snack. I assumed I had chronic low blood sugar, and even got tested for hypoglycemia and early-onset diabetes. (Both came back negative.) My doctor told me that everyone reacts differently to low levels of blood sugar, and I happened to be especially sensitive.

Then I did my Junk Cleanse (we're getting to it). After I finished, when I reincorporated real food back into my diet, I decided to rebuild my eating habits from scratch. This started with eggs. The first morning I scrambled two eggs, tossed in some cheese and salsa, and mixed it into a whole-wheat wrap. Delicious. By old conventional standards, since my new breakfast had 25 grams of fat, this should be more "fattening" than an entire week of low-fat cereal. But I didn't care; it was damn good. Then 10:30 a.m. rolled around, and instead of my usual hunger pangs, I felt fine. The next day I ate the same thing, and the next day I also felt fine. Light bulb moment. For nearly my entire adult life I thought I was hypoglycemic, but the truth is, I simply wasn't eating enough fat. Instead I was loading up on "healthy" cereal with a high dose of sugar. When the sugar crashed, so did I.

The eggs didn't make me any fatter. And I'm not alone. "In randomized and controlled trials, eating eggs results in more fat-loss and increased basal metabolism," argues Tim Ferriss in *The 4-Hour Body*. "In one such trial, overweight women who consumed a breakfast of two eggs a day for eight weeks (at least five days per week) instead of a bagel of equal weight and caloric value lost 65 percent more weight and—more important—had an 83 percent greater reduction in waist circumference."

Eggs are back.

Antibiotics in Red Meat

During my annual physical, I was chatting with my doctor about this book, and somehow the subject of antibiotics in meat came up. "Well, everybody knows *that's* bad for you," he says.

That's certainly the mainstream opinion. The debate over antibiotics has been raging since the Carter administration, with the meat industry saying that antibiotics are necessary to efficiently raise cattle, and health advocates charging that, essentially, they boost the resistance of bacteria, which poses a risk to us humans. Both sides seem to have a point. Since we tend to mostly hear from the antibiotics-are-evil camp—especially in the health community—I sought out a contrarian position.

Dr. Mike Apley is a professor of veterinary medicine at Kansas State University. He's also a cattle farmer. He writes articles for *Beef Magazine.* Far from the cliché you might expect of a Kansas cattleman, he's a scientist who speaks with authority on nutrition. "What you and I carry in our gut is certainly not isolated from what's in our food, and what's in our food is certainly not isolated from the environment and the animals," he tells me, acknowledging that there's a link, and therefore a risk, between the cattle's antibiotics and our bodies. But the question, as always, is degree. Dosage.

To put this risk in perspective, Apley explored the historic instances of food-borne illnesses carried by beef. "From 1998–2008, the CDC estimates there were 639,640 foodborne illnesses per year due to beef, including bacterial, chemical, and viral contamination," he writes in *Beef.* "We'll use this as our numerator. For a denominator, we'll take the low value of reported U.S. beef consumption from 2002 through 2008, which is 27 billion lbs. consumed. These data are available on the USDA Economic Research Service website."

His math is similar to my logic in the later section on salad, looking not just at the *relative* risk but also at the *absolute* risk. Yes, antibiotics-fed beef is probably riskier than grass-fed nonantibiotic beef, but by how much? Is the risk material? He continues, "Now we need to adjust for the amount of beef consumed per meal. It could be anything from 1-lb. steaks to the amounts contained in a beef hotdog or deli meat servings. If we pick .25 lb. as an average beef serving, that calculates to a total of 108 billion exposures per year. Our estimate of the number of beef-associated illnesses expressed as a percentage of beef 'exposures' is the product of 639,640 divided by 108 billion, which is 0.0000059. This can also be expressed as 0.0006 percent."

It's hard to fully appreciate the number 0.0006 percent, so Apley takes it one step further: "To look at it another way, during an average 80-year life expectancy, averaging 1 beef meal/day, that is 29,200 beef meals in a lifetime. Thus, our final estimate becomes one foodborne illness in six lifetimes."

Of course, there are plenty of reasons to eat grass-fed beef, and *less risk from foodborne illness* is just one of them. It might taste better. It might pack more nutritional punch. It might be better for the cattle and the environment. If you're concerned about the *risk of disease,* though, the antibiotics might be one less thing to worry about.

And then there's something else that's unfashionable to mention, but we should: Is it so wrong that we can produce beef economically? Doesn't that count for something? Imagine a world where the cost of beef triples. Yes, the vegetarians would have good reason to cheer, but what about the millions of lower- and middle-class Americans who, well, just want a damn hamburger?

"We aren't supposed to discuss this fact, but the food in this country is incredibly affordable," Apley tells me, noting that only 6 percent of Americans' income goes to food, compared to, say, 50 percent in Uganda. "We're a very well developed, sophisticated society where we have a whole lot of money to put minutes on the cell phone. But the reason we have so many other things . . . is that the foods we eat are so economical. Frankly, one of the emotions I see expressed—and I spend a lot of time with food-animal producers, is a kind of *amazement* of some of the attacks on modern agriculture. What we've done, I think, is provide a very safe, high-quality food source for the population."

This issue of antibiotics, fairly or not, reminds me of the no-MSG craze. And what happened to MSG, anyway?

MSG

A few years back, you couldn't go into a Chinese restaurant without hearing someone tell the waiter, "No MSG!" MSG, or monosodium glutamate, was the OG: original gluten.

Short version: That was all a bunch of hysteria. The only thing it did was put Chinese restaurants out of business.

As the FDA says:

"FDA considers the addition of MSG to foods to be 'generally recognized as safe' (GRAS). Although many people identify themselves as sensitive to MSG, in studies with such individuals given MSG or a placebo, scientists have not been able to consistently trigger reactions."

Or as food critic Jeffrey Steingarten asked, if MSG is really so evil, "why doesn't everyone in China have a headache?" There are fewer and fewer MSG studies (we've moved on to newer concerns, like gluten). "Scientific interest in its deleterious effects seems to be waning," notes the *Smithsonian*'s Natasha Geiling, as "the general scientific consensus seems to be that only in large doses and on an empty stomach can MSG temporarily affect a small subset of the population."

Yet again we freaked out for little reason.

Ice Cream

Okay, this one's a stretch. I confess that it took a *lot* of digging before I scrounged up any research that says we should eat more ice cream. It's true that in 2005, scientists conducted an experiment where people ate ice cream while having their brains scanned by MRIs (not at all awkward), demonstrating that the "pleasure centers" indeed light up when we eat ice cream. Afterward, someone involved with the study said, "This is the first time that we've been able to show that ice cream makes you happy. Just one spoonful lights up the happy zones of the brain in clinical trials." It's also true that the person who said this is a spokesperson for Unilever, which happens to own companies that make ice cream.*

But what if you're a woman who's trying to become pregnant?

---

*Just because something "lights up the happy zones of the brain" does not make it good for us. Something else that lights up the happy zone: cocaine.

Maybe you *should* eat ice cream. In 2007, Dr. Jorge Chavarro, a researcher at Harvard, concluded that low-fat dairy is more likely to lead to infertility than high-fat dairy. Women trying to conceive should "consider changing low-fat dairy foods for high-fat dairy foods; for instance, by swapping skimmed milk for whole milk and eating ice cream, not low-fat yogurt," according to Chavarro. Specifically, when analyzing the fertility rates and survey data of 18,555 women, after controlling for other variables (age, physical activity, weight, total calories consumed), he found that when women ate at least one high-fat source of dairy each day, they had a 27 percent lower risk of infertility. (The flip side: when women ate at least two servings of *low-fat* dairy, their risks of anovulatory infertility *increased* by 85 percent.) Yet another victory for fat.

There's even a book called *The Ice Cream Diet*. Then again it came out in 2002; is out of print; and is written by the same author as *The Peanut Butter Diet*. Let's just say it didn't take.

Carbs

"Fear of carbs, of gluten, of everything—we've distanced ourselves from the beauty of food, the art of it," says Olivia Wilde. "It makes me sad when people say, 'Oh, I don't eat gluten. I don't eat cheese. I don't eat this. So I eat cardboard.'"

She's got a point. People who say, "I can't eat that, it's got carbs!" are the world's most annoying dinner guests. (I say that as someone who's been that person.) But this isn't letting carbs off the hook. Too many carbs will make us fat. The supersizing of American bellies has a tidy correlation with the supersizing of refined carbohydrates; one in every three Americans is clinically obese (up from one in eight, in the 1960s), and we happen to eat a bajallion pounds of cheap bread and sugar. It's staggering.

As Gary Taubes argues in *Why We Get Fat,* there's not just a *link* between carbs and obesity, but a causal toppling of dominos: the very chemical makeup of carbohydrates spikes the level of our insulin, which makes us store fat. Even *thinking* about bagels can be fattening. "Because the insulin level in the bloodstream is determined primarily by the carbohydrates that are consumed . . . it's those carbohydrates that ultimately determine how much fat we accumulate," explains Taubes.

So what's the good news about carbs? Well, admittedly, not much. But according to other corners of the health industry, the pendulum has swung too far, and we now demonize carbs just as we used to demonize fat. The argument: Yes, it's true that when people reduce carbs they can reduce weight, but this is because they're reducing calories, period.

I spoke to carb defender Dr. Glenn Gaesser, director of the Healthy Lifestyles Research Center at ASU, chairman of the Grain Foods Foundation. "About half our calories comes from carbohydrates," he tells me. "One of the reasons that it has been successful to frame carbs as bad is that if you ask people to eliminate about half of what they eat, they will lose weight. It's an easy target. And it's easy to achieve a quick weight loss. The problem is, it's almost impossible to sustain." He cites studies showing that after one year, people on low-carb diets tend to regress back to their normal diet; meanwhile, the low-carb camp cites studies showing the opposite.

To oversimplify this, and to ensure that I offend every possible corner of the health industry:

Calories in, calories out! So says one camp. In this framework, carbs aren't necessarily all that bad, and you can have your bagel as long as you curb your overall caloric intake.

Not all calories are equal! So says the other camp. In this framework, they emphasize the glycemic index of certain foods, noting that sugars and breads will raise your insulin level, and this is what causes fat. You can eat as much meat and salad as you want without gaining weight.

Another charge against the low-carb camp: some nutritionists argue that it's ridiculous to obliterate an entire macronutrient from our diet. Just as there's good fat and bad fat, there are good carbs and bad carbs. Carrots have carbs. Broccoli has carbs. Should they be forbidden? "Lentils are a source of carbohydrates; they're a superfood. Lollipops are a source of carbohydrates; not so much. This focus on macro-nutrients is outdated nonsense." Dr. David Katz says on his blog. "Frankly, low-fat versus low-carb is just a bad question. What we care about is wholesome foods and sensible combinations."

I don't pretend to have the answer. I do have a bias toward moderation, so I'd like to believe that just as whiskey, steak, eggs, TV, stress, video games, and even bugs have merit in moderation, so, too, can grits and flapjacks. This works for millions of people. Then again, others find that carbs-in-moderation is nearly impossible, and for them, a policy of zero tolerance is the only way to drop weight.

How do we explain the fact that millions of people can eat bagels and not get fat? "A comparison with cigarettes is apt. Not every longtime smoker gets lung cancer. Only one in six men will, and one in nine women. But for those who do get lung cancer, cigarette smoke is far and away the most common cause," reasons

Taubes. "In a world without cigarettes, lung cancer would be a rare disease, as it once was. In a world without carbohydrate-rich diets, obesity would be a rare condition as well."

Because most of us grew up in the era of low fat, the concept of "carbs are fattening" seems a touch radical, untested, and dangerous. The Dietary Flavor of the Month. We think of the name "Atkins" and we grimace. But none of this, as Taubes freely admits, is anything new. The first serious low carber is likely eighteenth-century Jean Anthelme Brillat-Savarin, who published *The Physiology of Taste*, recommending that to avoid getting fat, people should cut down on "the starches and flours." The Banting Diet was born in 1862, when William Banting, who was obese, quickly shed thirty-five pounds by cutting "bread, butter, milk, sugar, beer, and potatoes," as he wrote in *Letter on Corpulence,* which tore up the bestseller lists. Taubes points out that in *Anna Karenina*, to stay lean, Count Vronsky "avoided starchy foods and desserts," and that in the next century, Saul Bellow's Herzog decides to not eat a candy bar, "thinking of the money he had spent on new clothes which would not fit if he ate carbohydrates." And on and on and on. Takeaway: The last fifty years that villainized fat are something of an extended aberration, *not* the original conventional wisdom. (Once again, we can thank Keys and the Food Pyramid.)

Maybe it's true that carbs are the primary agent responsible for weight gain. And maybe it's true that if I continue eating bagels and drinking beer I will never have a six-pack. I'm fine with that. I'm not giving up potatoes. As Taubes tells me on the phone, "It's as important to live well as it is to live long. If you're healthy, and happy, and you're eating carbs—there's an area where you can eat them in moderation." (Drink!)

Junk Food

It's time to put my money where my mouth is. Enough talk. We need action. For most of the book I've consulted with experts to explore the *theoretical* upside of bad things, but what happens when the rubber hits the road? How bad is bad?

One of the core principles in this book is that nothing, or almost nothing, is that bad for you in moderation. The real killer is dosage. So given that principle, I needed an experiment that would put it to the ultimate test: What if we took the crappiest food imaginable—food that no health expert would condone—and ate that, and only that, in moderation?

Or to look at it another way, in its simplest form, there are only two variables when it comes to food:

1. Quality of food
2. Quantity of food

We tend to think a lot about quality. We obsess about it. *Should we be eating organic or nonorganic? Grass-fed? Do I need to use whole grain pancake mix? Am I eating enough superfoods?* Concerns about the quality of food—fat versus carbs, processed versus unprocessed, our "macronutrient profile"—dominate the discussion. My experiment goes the other route. What happens when we ignore the quality of the food and focus only on the quantity?

So here's the game. For an entire month I would go on a junk food cleanse, which is identical to a juice cleanse, except that instead of drinking liquid kale I would eat Snickers, Doritos, and M&M's.

I would eat only four food groups:

1. Junk food
2. Black coffee
3. Protein shakes
4. Whiskey

I was inspired by a professor of nutrition at Kansas State University, Dr. Mark Haub, who, several years ago, as a demonstration for his class, put himself on a ten-week diet that was almost exclusively junk food, à la *Super Size Me*. He feasted on Twinkies, Oreos, and Little Debbies. Unlike Morgan Spurlock, he tracked his calories and capped his daily limit, careful to measure the portion size and eat everything in moderation. (We'll speak to him and hear his story in a bit. Dr. Haub deserves full credit as the architect of this experiment.)

These are the rules of the game: no vegetables, no fruit, no fresh meats or chicken or fish. No bread or pasta. Ideally my food should be able to be purchased in a gas station. (Dr. Haub's diet was also called the Gas Station Diet.) My friends also called it the Junk and Whiskey Cleanse or the "Snickers and Whiskey Diet." (I'm open to sponsorship.) No fast food, no pizza, no burgers, no fries: all too healthy. I only ate things that came wrapped in plastic.

Like Haub, I would meticulously count everything. I would track every calorie. This would be the ultimate test of calories in, calories out. I would eat whatever junk food I damn well pleased, but I capped my caloric intake at around 2,000, give or take, depending on physical activity. (The goal was to have a *net* caloric intake of 1,800, so I could eat 2,200 calories of Ho Hos if I burned 400 calories from a run.)

I went to my doctor's office immediately before the cleanse and immediately after for an official weigh-in. At six-foot-one I weighed in at 171 pounds, with a healthy cholesterol and blood profile.

Game on.

Day 1

Calories: 2,088
Exercise: 0

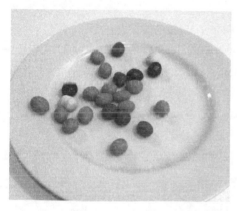

One serving size
of M&Ms

It didn't take long to feel the fatal flaw of this plan: the "serving size" of junk food is profoundly disappointing, and since I cap my portions to their official guidelines, I'm doomed to a month of 27 Cheez-Its and 3 Oreos. I counted every pretzel. I poured M&M's into measuring cups. I used a spreadsheet to allocate my junky calories throughout the day—150 calories of Oreos at 7:00 a.m., 200 calories of donuts at 9:00 a.m., etc. The math is ugly but it works. I was never exactly *hungry*, but I was never fully sated. One eye is always on the clock.

This is starting to feel like an awful idea.

Day 2

Calories: 2,426
Exercise: -475

I go for a run in the morning, popping a Little Debbie cake for pre-workout fuel. The run feels surprisingly good. *I* feel surprisingly good. Even though I hadn't had any honest-to-God food in twenty-four hours, it was comforting—even empowering—to know your body can come through in the clutch.

One good thing about junk food: it's super easy to track the calories. I use an app called My Fitness Pal, which has a barcode scanner, and since every candy bar has a barcode, you just zap the wrapper and the data is magically collected. This let me easily keep meticulous records.

Day 3

Calories: 2,152
Exercise: -428

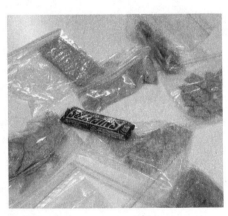

I prepared this in the morning every day

The cleanse is a pain in the ass. Measuring out portion size is easy when you're in the kitchen, but what if you're out and about, like I am today when touring Seattle with friends? I relied on Ziploc bags. In the morning I measured out exact portion sizes of Corn Nuts (⅓ cup), graham crackers (2 squares), donut holes (1 donut hole), protein powder (4 scoops), beef jerky (1 ounce), Hershey's chocolate bar, Snickers bar, Little Debbies, and I tossed it all in a backpack. My friend Cody calls this my "feast of shit."

Day 4
Calories: 1,690
Exercise: 0

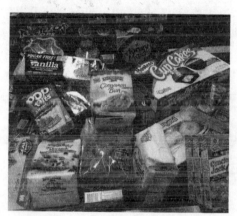

Grocery shopping

Grocery shopping time. I ignore my decade-long impulse to seek out "reduced fat," loading up the cart with full-fat Oreos, full-fat Chips Ahoy, and full-fat Doritos. I throw it all in the basket. The great thing about a junk cleanse is that there's no need to worry about buying too much, as nothing expires. (It's the Apocalypse Diet, as I could do it after civilization crumbles.)

A woman sees my cart and chuckles. "It looks amazing," she says. "That's all I'm craving, too."

I look up, see that she's pregnant. She has an excuse. What's mine?

Day 5

Calories: 2,365
Exercise: −330

"You're counting all the calories?" a friend asks.

"Every single one."

"But that's not really fair, is it?"

"Sure it's fair. It's my cleanse."

"But if you're eating fewer calories than you were before the cleanse, you don't know the true impact of junk food."

This is an important point. She's right to challenge me. The cleanse gives me a new appreciation for the thorniness of so many health studies, as I'm testing two variables at the same time:

Variable 1: Swapping real food for junk food
Variable 2: Lowering my calorie count

It's not a clean experiment. There's no way to know the true impact of junk food. Then again, that's not really the point. It's almost a certainty that, if I ate too much of it, junk food would be bad for me. That seems obvious. The more interesting question, for me, is what happens if I'm responsible about portion control (quantity) but irresponsible about the quality? *What we eat* versus *how much we eat.*

Day 6

Calories: 1,972
Exercise: −484

For breakfast, frozen Peanut M&M's. My body is adjusting. I've already made it longer than most "cleanses," which typically go just five days. In fact, the junk cleanse feels a lot like a juice cleanse. You're basically doing the same thing. Juicers tend to misdiagnose the reason they feel "lighter" or "cleansed"; they chalk it up to the magical power of "honey and cayenne pepper," but honey has nothing to do with it: you're starving your body of calories. You can do this with cayenne pepper or M&M's. I prefer candy.

Day 7
Calories: 2,195
Exercise: −392

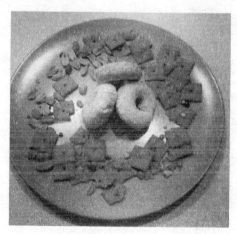

Breakthrough: junk food meals

A breakthrough day. Up until this point, I had been injecting calories linearly throughout the day, in even amounts, every hour or two. Starting today, I begin to clump these snacks in sad little meals, roughly corresponding to breakfast, lunch, and dinner. I have a supper of Chex mix, corn nuts, and Cracker Jack, anchored by a donut and sprinkled with Nerds, as a garnish.

Day 9
Calories: 2,240
Exercise: −446

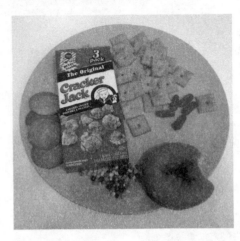

A fixture of many meals: Cracker Jack

For breakfast I enjoy a Little Debbie honey bun, taking the time to cut it with knife and fork to create the illusion that it's real food. Cracker Jack for dinner. Remember those "prizes" from Cracker Jack? I'm sad to report that they've seen better days; now it's just a lousy sticker. Or was it *always* a lousy sticker, and as we age we develop higher standards?

This whole operation wouldn't work without the protein shakes. They're crucial. But are they a cheat? I allow them because Dr. Haub, the godfather of the junk food cleanse, allowed them. As he told me, "A key tenet was to insure vitamin and mineral adequacy, thus, the protein shake." Since Haub is a responsible father, he also allowed himself a small portion of vegetables each day while at the dinner table (as an example for his kids) and then, after he left the table, he would consume his junk. I am not a father and I am not responsible, so I scotched the vegetables.

Day 11

Calories: 2,436
Exercise: −1,070

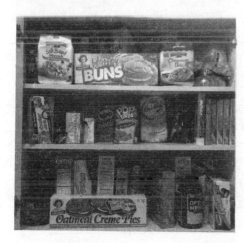

My new kitchen

I have a logistical problem. I live in New York, which means I have a kitchen the size of a bathtub, which means there's no room for all this junk food, as my cupboards are already stuffed with food-food. Something had to be done.

There's only one solution. In something of a cleansing ritual, I empty my cabinets of all real food. Pasta, rice vinegar, salt—no need for you. Gone. Olive oil, garlic powder, soy sauce—banished. I put all the food in deep storage. This cleaning ritual is the mirror image of what dieters do when they're told to only eat salads. It felt good. I stocked my now-empty cabinets with cookies and chips and candy.

Day 12

Calories: 3,116

Exercise: −189

Today I hit the U.S. Open. Muhammad Ali's daughter, Laila Ali, is a spokeswoman for USTA's tennis kids program, and I interview her for a potential story. She's teaming up with the USTA to battle obesity, and somehow my junk cleanse comes up.

"How do you *feel*?" she asks me.

"I feel fine,"

"Hmmmmmm." She clearly doesn't believe me. "Health is about more than skinny or fat," she says.

This is 100 percent true. My junk cleanse looks at the impact of junk food on *weight*, but it fails to measure all the intangible benefits of health, and there's no way for it to gauge the long-term impact. Yes, I feel surprisingly good after twelve days of eating garbage, but what's it doing to my cholesterol? My bones? My heart?

Day 13

Calories: 2,369

Exercise: −470

More Pop-Tarts, bourbon, and frozen ice-cream cones. I count out exactly 37 peanuts. This is a diet that no nutritionist would like. The low-fat wing would be appalled by my fat intake, courtesy of the candy bars, Doritos, and Little Debbies. The low-carbers would be shocked by the amount of refined sugars and carbs—Cheez-Its, corn chips, Nerds. The cleanse is not really low fat or low carb; it's just low IQ.

Day 14

Calories: 2,228

Exercise: -636

Date night. She didn't feel like drinking and I couldn't eat food, so we took a walk in a Brooklyn park, pretended we were fifteen years old, and went roller-skating. Eventually we end up at Shake Shack, where she ate a cheeseburger and I ate, well, nothing. Not at all emasculating.

Day 15

Calories: 2,497

Exercise: -406

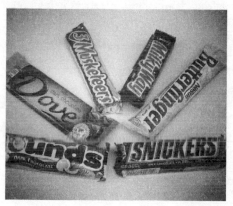

Variety is the spice of life

At the grocery store I buy a wider variety of candy bars, realizing my diet has been too monotonous. Why not experiment? I buy Dove, Mounds, Butterfinger. My godson asks me if I get a "cheat day" that lets me eat salad. Interesting idea, but I'm adamant: no real foods for a month.

Halfway there.

Day 18

Calories: 4,179

Exercise: 0

I decided to try a little experiment within the experiment. When you're on the "slow-carb" diet, Tim Ferriss recommends a weekly cheat day, where you go absolutely bat-shit crazy. This supposedly reboots the metabolism. So I do this, gorging myself on Ben and Jerry's ice cream, a king-size bag of corn chips, a king-size box of Hot Tamales, a dozen chocolate chip cookies, powdered donuts, and Little Debbie chocolate cupcakes. A total of 4,179 calories for the day.

I feel bloated, nauseous, sapped of energy. *This* is how people assumed I would feel. It's the junk cleanse without the portion control. *Shitty quality and too much quantity.* If I did *this* for thirty days, now we're talking Super Size Me. The scary thing is that it happened so naturally. It's easy to overeat. It's even easier to overeat with junk food. And it depressed me to realize that for much of America, this binge is just an average day.

Day 19

Calories: 2,123

Exercise: −533

A friend e-mails me an article: "The Secret to a Long Life? Fast Food." The founder of Chick-fil-A died at the age of ninety-three, leading *MarketWatch* to run a cheeky piece noting that fast-food moguls tend to have longer life spans:

- Irvine Robbins (Baskin Robbins), age 90
- Carl Karcher (Carl's Junior), age 89
- Ray Kroc (McDonald's), age 81

- Glen Bell (Taco Bell), age 86
- Wilber Hardee (Hardee's), age 89

See? Eat more junk food! (I'm sure the fact that these were billionaires had nothing to do with it. Example 547 of correlation versus causation.)

Day 21

Calories: 2,350

Exercise: -556

I've been eating beef jerky, which sparks intense debate among my friends. Does beef jerky count as junk food? Most agree that it does. It's sold in the junk food aisle, it's loaded with sodium, and it passes the one crucial test—you can buy it in a gas station. Others aren't convinced, reminding me that beef jerky, while gross, is still beef. This oddly parallels the real debates in the health community, such as whether tomato sauce on pizza should be classified as a vegetable. (Congress even passed a bill. Pizza's tomato sauce: vegetable.) My friend Cody comes down on me the hardest, saying, "A junk food cleanse is only as good as its integrity. And yours, sir, has none."

Day 22

Calories: 2,270

Exercise: -480

I wolf down an early dinner of corn chips, Cheez-Its, beef jerky, and Fig Newtons before I head to a restaurant for a date. She orders the fish; I order whiskey.

"You're not eating?" asks the waitress.

"I'm on a cleanse."

"But you can drink whiskey?"

'It's a new kind of cleanse."

(My date isn't quite sure what to think of this experiment. Or more to the point, she knows *exactly* what to think of it. A few weeks later she calls things off. But we can't be sure if this is correlation or causation.)

Day 23
Calories: 1,822
Exercise: 0

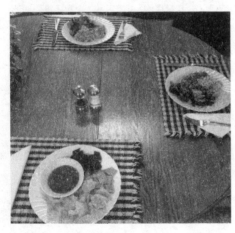

Family dinner

I visit my dad and stepmom. My stepmom is an excellent cook. She takes pride—and rightly so—in feeding the family food that is healthy and tasty. She catches wind of my little stunt and is worried about what to prepare.

"You guys just do your normal thing," I tell her. "I'm covered."

I show up at home with sacks of Doritos, corn chips, Cheez-Its, Pop-Tarts, beef jerky, and Cracker Jack. Her face is ashen. We sit down for family dinner. My dad and stepmom have plates of grilled salmon, steamed broccoli, and quinoa. I fix my own little plate of my feast of shit. It's a reminder that food is more than just fuel for the body—it's the backbone of social interaction. When you do weird things with food, you do weird things with your relationships.

Day 24

Calories: 1,967
Exercise: −453

"So your theory is that everything is okay in moderation, right?" asks my stepmom.

"Almost everything."

"So how do you eat a hamburger in moderation?"

I hadn't really considered that. With my typical unit of junk food, it's easy to dole out 27 Cheez-Its or 13 Doritos. But a burger? Who has the willpower to only eat *one-third* of a burger at a restaurant? This, of course, strikes at the profound unfairness of body type; restaurants serve everyone the same amount of calories per burger, whether you weigh 110 or 210 pounds. Calories in, calories out can be cruel math.

Day 26

Calories: 1,786
Exercise: 0

Today I get my hair cut. I tell my barber, a little too proudly, "I haven't had any fruit, vegetables, meat, or bread in twenty-five days."

"I can tell. Your hair is thinner."

Really?

"Yeah, normally I'm on the fence as to whether I need to use my thinning scissors, but this time, it's a no-brainer. I don't need them."

"It's thin everywhere?"

"Everywhere. You need that food, man. You need the nutrients."

He looks at my eyebrows, which he once described as the fastest-growing eyebrows he's seen in his career. "Even your eyebrows have suffered. They're weak." I sink lower in my chair.

It's an important reminder. What else is wrong with my body that I can't detect?

Assessing health isn't as simple as just reading the numbers on a scale, or even the cholesterol readings. Our bodies are infinitely nuanced and subtle. If it's true that my hair is thinning, who knows how this diet of junk is affecting my skin, bones, or testosterone levels? What if my future kids have Snickers in their blood?

My barber inspects my head. "On the bright side, your ear hair is still growing."

Day 27

Calories: 2,074

Exercise: -408

I chat with Nina Teicholz, author of *The Big Fat Surprise*. We discuss her book and mine, and I mention the absurdity of my junk cleanse. She's a good sport and she considers it. "Our bodies are really good at storing nutrients," she tells me. "You have plenty of nutrients stored from years of healthier eating." So she's not surprised that I'm feeling okay after just a few weeks of shitty eating; like others, she points out that, hypothetically, if I continued on this path for a year or five years or ten years, it would likely be a different story.

Day 29

Calories: 2,481

Exercise: -427

Three Oreos for breakfast. And I feel fine. Why is that? Let's compare the nutritional content of Oreos to the nutritional content of my usual breakfast:

3 Oreos
Calories: 200
Fat: 9.3 grams
Carbs: 33.3 grams
Sugar: 18.7 grams
Protein: 1.3 grams
Vitamins A and C: 0
Calcium: 0
Iron: 10.7 percent
Dietary fiber: 1 gram

Trader Joe's Frosted Maple & Brown Sugar Shredded Wheat
Technically a serving size is 1 cup, but I tend to have about 1.5 cups, so we'll use that:

Calories: 300
Fat: 1.5 grams
Carbs: 63 grams
Sugar: 18 grams
Protein: 7.5 grams
Vitamins A and C: 0
Calcium: 0
Iron: 135 percent
Dietary fiber: 7.5 grams

My usual cereal is typically thought of as "healthy." It's not Cocoa Puffs or Froot Loops; the cover of the box features wholesome looking grains and cantaloupe. But if we peel away the labels and the baggage, how much difference is there between this cereal and three Oreos? Yes, it has more protein and fiber— and that's important—but there's just as much sugar and twice as many carbs. This isn't to praise the virtue of Oreos, but to question the merits of "healthy" food. (More on this in the flip side of the book.)

Day 30
Calories: 1,827
Exercise: −381

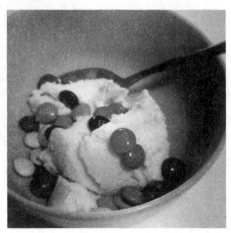

A well-balanced diet

I discover the joy of sugar-free Jell-O. It's like cheating! You can devour an entire tub and it only costs 40 calories. (For the moment, I'll ignore the recent evidence saying artificial sweeteners are bad for you.)

I'm close to the end. People are asking me what I crave. Salad? A burger?

I crave more junk food. I have something like Stockholm syndrome, as the sugary snacks have kidnapped me. I have become afraid of real food. For this we can thank the brilliant engineers at Nabisco, Kraft, General Mills, et al., who, after spending millions on R&D, carefully calibrate the sugars in their food to the optimal "bliss point" to make it addictive. For a month I've been eating nothing but the Bliss Point. And I want more.

Although, when I confess to my mom that I'm not craving salad, she brings up a good point. "Jeff, *no one* has ever craved salad."

Day 31
Calories: 2,311
Exercise: −515

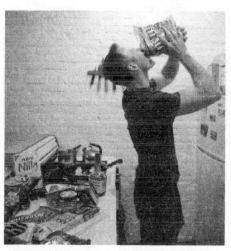

Breakfast

Someone forwards me an article from *Men's Health*: "A Day Spent Eating Nothing But Dark Chocolate," subtitled, "Would this be cacao heaven or hell? The author soon found out."

Rookie, please. Talk to me in a month.

Day 33

Calories: 2,994

Exercise: −427

I've done it. Mission accomplished.

I head to the doctor's office for my blood work and official weigh-in.

I step on the scale. My doctor fiddles with the scale, frowns, looks at the clipboard, then looks back at the scale. He makes an adjustment.

"Huh," he says.

Good huh or bad huh?

"You lost eleven pounds, he says, double-checking his notes.

Jesus. I had suspected I'd lose weight—calories in, calories out—but I didn't think it would be that dramatic.

"Eleven pounds in a month. That's *not healthy*," he says. "No one should lose that much weight so quickly."

Of course he's right. This is not a diet or a plan that I recommend. And what about the blood work and the cholesterol?

There were a few changes. . . .

My bad cholesterol: went down.

My good cholesterol: went up.

Everything else stayed the same or had a mild improvement. My body fat dipped by about two percentage points.

Remember Dr. Mark Haub, my inspiration for the cleanse? He lost twenty-seven pounds in ten weeks. (No word on how much hair.)

How is this possible? Calories in, calories out. This is no longer a fashionable maxim, as we're obsessed with parsing "good fats" from "bad fats" and "good carbs" from "bad carbs." Which isn't wrong. But it tends to make dietary guidelines confusing as hell, so Haub wanted to prove that at the end of the day, to lose weight, it's all about *consuming less than you burn*—no matter what you eat.

He's quick to agree that, yes, of course, not all calories have the same impact on our bodies: 50 calories of almonds will be digested differently than 50 calories of sugar. "But from a larger picture, we're getting confused," he tells me. "The laws of thermodynamics still hold true. Energy in, energy out. And I wanted to be a guinea pig to prove that."

This scandalized the health community. After CNN announced that the "Twinkie diet helps nutrition professor lose 27 pounds," soon other health experts condemned the experiment and argued that, yes, he lost weight, but you can also lose weight by getting cancer or wasting away from AIDS. The Mayo Clinic frowned upon the Twinkie diet, advising, "It's anything but balanced. His food choices leave much to be desired. Carbs are mostly sugar. [His] saturated fat is double that recommended by experts."

"People were looking for excuses, because the diet didn't comport to their understanding. They were poking around to find something that's not healthy," says Haub.

But they couldn't find anything. Not only did he lose weight, but his LDL (bad cholesterol) dropped 20 percent. His body mass index plunged from 28.8 to 24.9—overweight to normal. Haub seems to relish challenging the status quo—even his Twitter bio reads "Favor science-based wisdom over conventional."

"A lot of physicians painted themselves in a corner," Haub tells me. "They say that because I did it the *wrong* way, it's not healthy.

But how are we defining health? Isn't it healthier to not be over-weight? And I did it through eating junk food."

Some experts weren't that shocked at the outcome. You'll recognize one of them. "We've made altogether too much over fat versus carbs and it's a huge distraction for the most part," said Dr. Katz. "The fundamental truth is that at energy balance, calories in versus calories used determines weight, and this reinforces that." (Katz also points out that it's hard to "feel full" on the empty calories of Twinkies, so this is unlikely to be a long-term solution. After doing it for a month, I would agree.)

After I finished my own junk cleanse I e-mailed Haub and told him the results. He suspected people would again dismiss the experiment, saying "It's only a sample size of one."

Well, now we have a sample size of two.

So how does this square with the growing body of research that says the real enemy is carbs? It's possible that even though cheap carbs and sugars made up a dizzying percentage of my diet, my *overall intake of food* was lower than usual, so my carb intake was still reduced. I didn't lose weight because I ate more carbs; I lost weight because I consumed less food. The results would almost as-suredly have been better if, instead of allocating these 2,000 calories willy-nilly among cheap junk food, I instead consumed 2,000 calories of plants, protein, and fat.

Another takeaway: tracking is helpful. It keeps you honest. Tim Ferriss suggests the same thing. "Nonconsistent tracking equals no awareness equals no behavioral change. Consistent tracking, even if you have no knowledge of fat loss or exercise, will often beat advice from world-class trainers."

The point isn't that junk food is good. It's not. And of course if I had eaten all this garbage *on top* of my normal diet, as opposed to a *replacement* of my normal diet, I would have ballooned. The point is that moderation is such a powerful force that it works *even when you're eating crap.*

The crap isn't the enemy.

Excess is the enemy.

Final Thoughts

We like to judge. It's what humans do. If a guy says his favorite band is Nickelback, we judge him to have bad taste. Health is no different. A certain corner of society has become so pious about health, so sanctimonious, that they judge others for eating beef, choosing not to buy organic, or shrugging about things like GMOs and BPA. I'm guilty of judging and I'm guilty of being judged. It lets us feel better about ourselves. (*At least I'm not as bad as That Guy.*) It'd be one thing if the science supports that judgment. But sometimes it doesn't. The link between many of these "bad things" and "bad health" is, at best, questionable. Drinkers tend to live longer than nondrinkers. Red meat is not a killer. Even eating *dirt* might not be so bad for you.

This has implications. If you think of yourself as relatively healthy, but you worry that you're "not doing enough" or eating the "right foods," the good news is that you might be just fine. Results trump method. If you barely pay attention to what you eat, but somehow you have good blood pressure, you feel healthy, and the doctor pronounces you fit, then why beat yourself up?

Or maybe, like many of us, you *don't* feel fine. What if you feel sluggish and want to drop a few pounds, lower your cholesterol, start an exercise program? Excellent. Now you've seen that—according to gobs of studies and a growing wing of the health community—the best way to lose that weight might *not* be to go low-fat, but instead to eat a variety of foods and focus on portion control. *How much* you eat is just as important as what you eat—maybe even more important. Don't demonize food. Demonize excess.

And don't get distracted by all the whiplash from health news. So much of it is just noise. The biggest misconception about health, according to Dr. Katz, is that "what we need to know about diet is something that we haven't figured out yet. We're waiting for tomorrow's epiphany. There will be no epiphany tomorrow. We already know everything we need to know to eliminate virtually all obesity and almost all diet-related disease; we just don't do it. We don't do it because it involves actual effort."

This might seem contrary to the spirit of the book—good news about what's bad, bad news about what's good—but I view it as consistent. *Beneath all the news* is a set of core principles: eat food in moderation, exercise in moderation, goof off in moderation. This allows plenty of wiggle room for things like naps and tequila. Socrates with his Greek Golden Mean, once again, has the last laugh.

Let's leave this section on a hopeful note. There's one more health study you should know about: In October 2014, the CDC announced that, for Americans, the average life expectancy reached an all-time high of 78.8 years—81.2 for women, 76.4 for men. So even with all the doom and gloom stories about how we're all so fat and lazy, somehow, we're living longer.

That's good news, right?

I'm off to grab a whiskey.

Sources

One thing is abundantly clear: This book couldn't have been written without the invaluable resources—and archives—of news outlets like *The New York Times*, *The Washington Post*, *Slate*, and *Scientific American*. The *Times'* "Well Blog," in particular, was a godsend. A journalist thanking *The New York Times* is like a swimmer thanking water—there's a reason it pops up again and again in the text. Thank you to all of the countless researchers, journalists, and editors who continue to add to our body of health knowledge.

INTERVIEWS

The following were interviewed by telephone, e-mail, or in person:

Alison Van Eenennaam, by telephone, July 25, 2014
Barry Schwartz, by telephone, August 19, 2014
Brett Ford, by e-mail, August 22, 2014
Carl Lavie, by e-mail, August 9, 2014
Cody Dolan, by e-mail, September 19, 2014
David J. Hanson, by telephone, April 15, 2014
David Katz, by telephone, June 4, 2014

David Katz, video blog, September 25, 2014

David Ley, by e-mail, July 18, 2014

David Marcus, by telephone, June 9, 2014

David Ropeik, by telephone, September 4, 2014

David Tovey, by telephone, October 28, 2014

Don J. Q. Chen, by e-mail, August 8, 2014

Frank Partnoy, by telephone, August 8, 2014

Gary Taubes, by telephone, September 10, 2014

Glenn Gaesser, by telephone, September 4, 2014

Gloria Brame, by e-mail, July 31, 2014

Guy Winch, by telephone, April 18, 2014

Ivan Oransky, by telephone, April 29, 2015

Jeffrey Rubin, by telephone, June 12, 2014

Jodi Gilman, by e-mail, August 26, 2014

Jonathan Berman, by e-mail, August 21, 2014

Katherine Beals, by e-mail, June 25, 2014

Laila Ali, in-person, September 1, 2014

Mark Haub, by telephone, May 15, 2014

Maryka Quik, by telephone, July 25, 2014

Michael Apley, by telephone, September 26, 2014

Michael Cunningham, by telephone, April 4, 2014

Nina Teicholz, by telephone, September 4, 2014

Phil Torres, by e-mail, August 14, 2014

Rachel Neale, by e-mail, August 30, 2014

Richard Stack, by telephone, July 8, 2013

Richard Stephens, by telephone, June 12, 2014

Robert London, by telephone, April 21, 2014

Robin Kowalski, by telephone, April 9, 2014

Ruslan Medzhitov, by telephone, September 11, 2014

Sera Young, by telephone, July 15, 2014

Shelley Case, by telephone, September 11, 2014

Stuart Lewis, in-person, September 22, 2014

Thomas Dunn, telephone, March 13, 2015

Valerie Curtis, by telephone, June 13, 2014

Introduction

Mark Bittman, "Butter Is Back," *New York Times*, March 25, 2014.

A. J. Jacobs, *Drop Dead Healthy: One Man's Humble Quest for Bodily Perfection*, Simon & Schuster, 2012.

Ron Rosenbaum, "Let Them Eat Fat," *Wall Street Journal*, March 15, 2013.

FOOD
Fat

Allison Aubrey, "Cutting Back on Carbs, Not Fat, May Lead to More Weight Loss," NPR, September 1, 2014.

L. Hooper et al., "Dietary Fat Intake and Prevention of Cardiovascular Disease: Systematic Review," *British Medical Journal* 322, no. 7289 (2001): 757–763.

"Fats and Cholesterol: Out with the Bad, In with the Good," *The Nutrition Source*, Harvard School of Public Health, www.hsph.harvard.edu/nutritionsource /fats-full-story/; accessed November 15, 2014.

Michael F. Roizen, "Diet, Diet on the Wall, Which Is the Healthiest of Them All?" *U.S. News and World Report*, September 11, 2014.

Gary Taubes, *Why We Get Fat: And What to Do About It*, Anchor, 2011.

Nina Teicholz, *The Big Fat Surprise: Why Butter, Meat and Cheese Belong in a Healthy Diet*, Simon & Schuster, 2014.

Nina Teicholz, "The Last Anti-Fat Crusaders," *Wall Street Journal*, October 28, 2014.

Bryan Walsh, "Ending the War on Fat," *Time*, June 12, 2014.

Gluten

Karen Ansel, "Is Gluten Bad for You?" *Women's Health*, November 6, 2010.

Jane Brody, "Celiac Disease, a Common, but Elusive, Diagnosis," *New York Times*, September 29, 2014.

Luisa Dillner, "Is Gluten Bad for Your Health?" *Guardian*, August 25, 2014.

Sydney Lupkin, "5 Gluten Myths You Were Too Embarrassed to Ask About," ABCNews.com, May 9, 2014.

Michael Specter, "Against the Grain," *New Yorker*, November 3, 2014.

Stephanie Strom, "A Big Bet on Gluten-Free," *New York Times*, February 17, 2014.

Salt

Aaron Carroll, "Dash of Salt Does No Harm. Extremes Are the Enemy," *New York Times*, August 25, 2014.

N. A. Graudal, T. Hubeck-Graudal, and G. Jurgens, "Effects of Low Sodium Diet Versus High Sodium Diet on Blood Pressure, Renin, Aldosterone, Catecholamines, Cholesterol, and Triglyceride," *Cochrane Database System Review*, November 9, 2011, doi: 10.1002/14651858.CD004022. pub3.

"Why Salt May Not Be So Bad for You After All," *Economist*, April 28, 2014.

Gary Taubes, "Salt, We Misjudged You," *New York Times*, June 12, 2012.

Chocolate

Roger Dobson, "Love Long and Eat Chocolate," *Sydney Morning Herald*, December 15, 2008.

U. Heinrich et al., "Long-Term Ingestion of High Flavanol Cocoa Provides Photoprotection Against UV-Induced Erythema and Improves Skin Condition in Women." *Journal of Nutrition*, 2006 Jun;136(6):1565-9. PMID: 16702322

Alok Jha, "Chocolate Reduces Stroke Risk for Men, Research Claims," *Guardian*, August 30, 2012.

Gretchen Reynolds, "Why Chocolate Is Good for Us," *New York Times*, April 24, 2014.

Mauro Serafini et al., "Plasma Antioxidants from Chocolate," *Nature*, August 28, 2003.

GMOs

Molly Ball, "Want to Know If Your Food Is Genetically Modified?" *Atlantic*, May 14, 2014.

Drake Bennett, "Inside Monsanto, America's Third-Most-Hated Company," *Businessweek,* July 3, 2014.

Amy Harmon, "A Lonely Quest for Facts on Genetically Modified Crops," *New York Times*, January 4, 2014.

Mark Lynas, "How I Got Converted to G.M.O. Food," *New York Times*, April 24, 2015.

Tamar Haspel, "The GMO Debate: 5 Things to Stop Arguing," *Washington Post*, October 27, 2014.

C. Snell et al., "Assessment of the Health Impact of GM Plant Diets in Long-Term and Multigenerational Animal Feeding Trials: A Literature Review," *Food Chemistry and Toxicology*, March 2012, PMID: 22155268.

McDonald's

John Cisna, *My McDonald's Diet*, Instinct Media, LLC, 2014.

Samantha Grossman, "Teacher Loses 37 Pounds After Three-Month McDonald's Diet," Time.com, January 5, 2014. http://newsfeed.time.com/2014/01/05/teacher-loses-37-pounds-after-three-month-mcdonalds-diet/

Katherine Klingseis, "McDonald's Diet Leaves Iowa Teacher 61 Pounds Lighter," *Des Moines Register*, March 18, 2014.

DRINK
Bourbon

Auslan Cramb, "Whisky 'Helps Fight Cancer,'" *Telegraph*, May 9, 2005.

Sanjay Gupta, "Work Out and Drink Up," *Time*, January 17, 2008.

Stanton Peele, "The Truth We Won't Admit: Drinking Is Healthy," *Pacific Standard*, August 12, 2014.

Coffee

Neal D. Freedman, "Association of Coffee Drinking with Total and Cause-Specific Mortality," *New England Journal of Medicine*, May 7, 2012.

Latarsha Gatlin, "Caffeine Has Positive Effect on Memory, Johns Hopkins Researchers Say," JHU.edu, January 12, 2014. http://hub.jhu.edu/2014/01/12/caffeine-enhances-memory

Donald Hensrud, "Is Coffee Good or Bad for Me?" MayoClinic.com, March 13, 2014. www.mayoclinic.org/healthy-living/nutrition-and-healthy-eating/expert-answers/coffee-and-health/faq-20058339

Rachel Nuwer, "For Truck Drivers, Coffee May Save Lives," *Smithsonian*, March 21, 2013.

Beer

Jeanna Bryner, "Beer May Be Good for Your Bones," LiveScience.com, February 7, 2010. www.livescience.com/6072-beer-good-bones.html

Rob Stein, "Daily Drink Helps Keep Brain Sharp, Data Suggest," *Washington Post*, January 20, 2005.

Drinking During Pregnancy

"Alcohol Use in Pregnancy," Centers for Disease Control and Prevention, CDC
.gov, accessed August 1, 2014. www.cdc.gov/ncbddd/fasd/alcohol-use.html

"BJOG study: Light Drinking During Pregnancy Is Not Linked to Adverse Be-
havioural or Cognitive Outcomes in Childhood," BJOG.org, April 17, 2013.
www.bjog.org/details/news/4608611/BJOG_study_Light_drinking_during
_pregnancy_is_not_linked_to_adverse_behavioural_.html

Meghan Holohan, "New Study Shows No Harm from Moderate Drinking in
Pregnancy, But Experts Urge Caution," Today.com, January 3, 2014. www
.today.com/parents/new-study-shows-no-harm-moderate-drinking
-pregnancy-experts-urge-2D11849699

Mayo Clinic Staff, "Pregnancy Nutrition: Foods to Avoid During Pregnancy,"
MayoClinic.com, September 4, 2014. www.mayoclinic.org/healthy-living
/pregnancy-week-by-week/in-depth/pregnancy-nutrition/art-20043844

Anne-Marie Nybo Andersen et al., "Moderate Alcohol Intake During Pregnancy
and Risk of Fetal Death," *Oxford University Press*, October 27, 2011.

Emily Oster, "I Wrote That It's OK to Drink While Pregnant. Everyone Freaked
Out. Here's Why I'm Right," *Slate*, September 11, 2013.

Tequila

Melanie Haiken, "New Sweetener from the Tequila Plant May Aid Diabetes,
Weight Loss," *Forbes*, March 17, 2014.

Christine Hsu, "Drinking Alcohol May Significantly Enhance Problem Solving
Skills," MedicalDaily.com, April 11, 2012. www.medicaldaily.com/drinking
-alcohol-may-significantly-enhance-problem-solving-skills-240105

Red Wine

Sam Dean, "Is Wine Good for You? Or Bad? What Does Science Say?" *Bon
Appétit*, July 11, 2014.

Kim Edwards, "A Modest Glass of Wine Each Day Could Improve Liver Health,"
UC San Diego News Center, May 19, 2008.

"How Red Wine May Shield Brain from Stroke Damage," HopkinsMedicine.org,
April 21, 2010. www.hopkinsmedicine.org/news/media/releases/How_Red
_Wine_May_Shield_Brain_From_Stroke_Damage

BAD HABITS
Profanity

Foster Kamer, "'Fuck,' Carol Bartz: A Brief History of Yahoo's Ousted CEO and Bad Words," *New York Observer*, September 8, 2011.

Louise Tickle, "Research Demonstrates How the Use of Bad Language Can Alter Our Behavior," *Guardian*, October 3, 2011.

Jennifer Waters, "What the Bleep? Swearing at Work Can Inspire Teamwork," *MarketWatch*, October 18, 2007.

Messiness

Eric Abrahamson, *A Perfect Mess: The Hidden Benefits of Disorder. How Crammed Closets, Cluttered Offices, and on-the-Fly Planning Make the World a Better Place*, Little, Brown, 2007.

Ilan Mochari, "The Psychology of Messiness: How Disorder Can Make You More Creative," *Inc.*, April 2, 2014.

Kathleen Vohs, "It's Not 'Mess.' It's Creativity," *New York Times*, September 13, 2013.

Napping

Eric Barker, "Why You Should Really Take a Nap This Afternoon, According to Science," *The Week*, July 25, 2014.

Charles E. Basch et al., "Prevalence of Sleep Duration on an Average School Night Among 4 Nationally Representative Successive Samples of American High School Students, 2007–2013," Centers for Disease Control, 2014.

Colin D. Chapman et al, "Acute Sleep Deprivation Increases Food Purchasing in Men," *Obesity*, September 5, 2013.

Tara Parker-Pope, "Lost Sleep Can Lead to Weight Gain," *New York Times*, March 18, 2013.

"Penn Medicine Researchers Show How Lost Sleep Leads to Lost Neurons," UPenn.edu (Perelman School of Medicine), March 18, 2014.

Fidgeting

Nick Collins, "Fidgeting Could Prolong Your Life," *Telegraph*, June 29, 2012.

K. Ashlee McGuire and Robert Ross, "Incidental Physical Activity Is Positively

Associated with Cardiorespiratory Fitness," *Medicine & Science in Sports & Exercise* 2011, doi: 10.1249.

Mary Murphy, "Obesity Expert Says Daily Workouts Can't Undo Damage Done from Sitting All Day," *NBCNews.com*, January 9, 2013. http://rockcenter .nbcnews.com/_news/2013/01/09/16431050-obesity-expert-says-daily -workouts-cant-undo-damage-done-from-sitting-all-day?lite

Gretchen Reynolds, "Fidgeting Your Way to Fitness," *New York Times*, May 11, 2011.

Complaining

Guy Winch, *The Squeaky Wheel: Complaining the Right Way to Get Results, Improve Your Relationships, and Enhance Self-Esteem*, Walker, 2011.

Gossip

Robin Dunbar, *Grooming, Gossip, and the Evolution of Language*, Harvard University Press, 1998.

"Gossip and Ostracism May Have Hidden Group Benefits," *PsychologicalScience .org*, January 27, 2014. www.psychologicalscience.org/index.php/news /releases/gossip-and-ostracism-may-have-hidden-group-benefits.html

Alina Tugend, "Studies Find That Gossip Isn't Just Loose Talk," *New York Times*, June 15, 2012.

Laziness

Eh.

Procrastination

Frank Partnoy, *Wait: The Art and Science of Delay*, PublicAffairs, 2013.

VICE AND DIVERSIONS
Nicotine

Dan Hurley, "Will a Nicotine Patch Make You Smarter?" *Scientific American*, February 9, 2014.

Nancy Humphrey, "Nicotine May Aid Memory for Some Older Adults: Study," News.Vanderbilt.edu, January 13, 2012. http://news.vanderbilt.edu/2012/01 /nicotine-may-aid-memory-for-some-older-adults-study/

Kristen Philipkoski, "Study: Nicotine Is Good for You," Gizmodo.com, January 10, 2012. http://gizmodo.com/5874885/study-nicotine-is-good-for-you

Pot

Brian Palmer, "How Bad Is Marijuana for Your Health?" *Slate*, May 1, 2014.

Scott Rappold, "Legalize Medical Marijuana, Doctors Say in Survey," WebMD.com, April 2, 2014. www.webmd.com/news/breaking-news/marijuana-on-main-street/20140225/webmd-marijuana-survey-web

Abigail Sullivan Moore, "This is Your Brain on Drugs," *New York Times*, October 29, 2014.

Maia Szalavitz, "Is Marijuana Addictive? It Depends How You Define Addiction," *Time*, October 19, 2010.

Video Games

Linda Carroll, "Video Games Are Good for You (A Little Bit)," Today.com, August 4, 2014. www.today.com/health/video-games-are-good-you-little-bit 1D80005579

Children's Health Team, "Active Gaming May Help Your Child Lose Weight," *Cleveland Clinic*, April 10, 2014.

Nic Fleming, "Why Video Games May Be Good for You," BBC.com, August 26, 2013. www.bbc.com/future/story/20130826-can-video-games-be-good-for-you

D. Giannotti et al., "Play to Become a Surgeon: Impact of Nintendo Wii Training on Laparoscopic Skills," PLoS One, 2013, PMID: 23460845.

Laura Kurtzman, "Training the Older Brain in 3-D: Video Game Enhances Cognitive Control," UCSF.edu, September 4, 2013. https://www.ucsf.edu/news/2013/09/108616/training-older-brain-3-d-video-game-enhances-cognitive-control

Joseph Nordqvist, "Tetris Video Game Helps Treat Lazy Eye," *Medical News Today*, April 23, 2013. www.medicalnewstoday.com/articles/259547.php

Web Surfing

Rachel Emma Silverman, "Web Surfing Helps at Work, Study Says," *Wall Street Journal*, August 22, 2011.

Porn

David Ley, Nicole Prause, and Peter Finn, "The Emperor Has No Clothes: A Review of the 'Pornography Addiction' Model," *Current Sexual Health Reports*, February 12, 2014.

Melinda Wenner Moyer, "The Sunny Side of Smut," *Scientific American*, June 23, 2011.

Gad Saad, "Pornography: Beneficial or Detrimental?" *Psychology Today*, January 22, 2010.

Pornhub.com FOR RESEARCH ONLY.

Masturbation

Michael Castleman, "How Common Is Masturbation, Really?" *Psychology Today*, March 30, 2009.

"92 percent of Women Are Regularly 'Pleasing Themselves,'" SourceWire.com, December 11, 2008. www.sourcewire.com/news/44083/92-of-women-are-regularly-pleasing-themselves-#.VUfqtc7008I

TV

Jaye L. Derrick, "Energized by Television: Familiar Fictional Worlds Restore Self-Control," *Social Psychological and Personality Science*, May 2013.

Steven Johnson, *Everything Bad Is Good for You: How Today's Popular Culture Is Actually Making Us Smarter*, Riverhead Trade, 2006.

Ecstasy

John H. Halpern et al., "Residual Neurocognitive Features of Long-Term Ecstasy Users with Minimal Exposure to Other Drugs," *Addiction*, April 2011, doi: 10.1111/j.1360-0443.2010.03252.x.

Robin McKie, "Ecstasy Does Not Wreck the Mind, Study Claims," *Guardian*, February 19, 2011.

David Nutt, *Drugs Without the Hot Air*, UIT Cambridge Ltd, 2012.

David J. Nutt, Leslie A. King, and Lawrence D. Phillips, "Drug Harms in the UK: A Multicriteria Decision Analysis," *Lancet*, November 6, 2010, doi:10.1016/S0140-6736(10)61462-6.

BAD MIND-SETS
Stress
Centre for Studies on Human Stress, "Biology of Stress," HumanStress.ca.

A. Keller et al., "Does the Perception That Stress Affects Health Matter? The Association with Health and Mortality," *Health Psychology* 31, no. 5 (2012): 677–684.

Kelly McGonigal, "How to Make Stress Your Friend," TED Talk, June 2013.

Jane Weaver, "Can Stress Actually Be Good For You?" NBCNews.com, December 20, 2006. www.nbcnews.com/id/15818153/ns/health-mental_health/t/can-stress-actually-be-good-you/

Introversion
Susan Cain, *Quiet: The Power of Introverts in a World That Can't Stop Talking*, Broadway Books, 2013.

Jennifer Kahnweiler, *Quiet Influence: The Introvert's Guide to Making a Difference*, Berrett-Koehler Publishers, 2013.

Selfishness
Jonathan Berman and Deborah Small, "Self-Interest Without Selfishness: The Hedonic Benefit of Imposed Self-Interest," *Psychological Science*, September 10, 2012, doi: 10.1177/0956797612441222.

Disgust
Valerie Curtis, *Don't Look, Don't Touch, Don't Eat: The Science Behind Revulsion*, University of Chicago Press, 2013.

James Gorman, "Survival's Ick Factor," *New York Times*, January 23, 2012.

Failure
Costica Bradatan, "In Praise of Failure," *New York Times*, December 15, 2013.

Worrying
Steven Berglas, "Worried About Anxiety? Don't Be; It's Often Good For You," *Forbes*, January 25, 2013.

Suzanne R. Dash, Frances Meeten, and Graham C. L. Davey, "Systematic Information Processing Style and Perseverative Worry," *Clinical Psychology Review*, December 2013.

"Excessive Worrying May Have Co-evolved with Intelligence," SUNY Down-state Medical Center, Downstate.edu, April 13, 2012.

Spite

Natalie Angier, "Spite Is Good. Spite Works," *New York Times*, March 31, 2014.

"In Sex, Happiness Hinges on Keeping Up with the Joneses, CU-Boulder Study Finds," University of Colorado Boulder, Colorado.edu, April 15, 2013. www.colorado.edu/news/releases/2013/04/15/sex-happiness-hinges-keeping-joneses-cu-boulder-study-finds

D. K. Marcus et al., "The Psychology of Spite and the Measurement of Spite-fulness," *Psychological Assessment,* February 17, 2014, dx.doi.org/10.1037/a0036039.

Anger

Brett Ford and Iris Mauss, "The Paradoxical Effects of Pursuing Positive Emo-tion: When and Why Wanting to Feel Happy Backfires," in *Positive Emotion: Integrating the Light Sides and Dark Sides*, edited by June Gruber and Judith Tedlie Moskowitz, Oxford University Press, 2014.

Yoda, *Star Wars, Episode I: The Phantom Menace*, 1999.

(ALMOST) EVERYTHING ELSE
Obesity

Harriet Brown, "In 'Obesity Paradox,' Thinner May Mean Sicker," *New York Times*, September 17, 2012.

Carl Lavie, *The Obesity Paradox: When Thinner Means Sicker and Heavier Means Healthier*, Hudson Street Press, 2014.

Dirt

Sera Young, *Craving Earth: Understanding Pica: The Urge to Eat Clay, Starch, Ice, and Chalk,* Columbia University Press, 2012.

Pesticides

Dena Bravata et al., "Are Organic Foods Safer or Healthier than Conven-tional Alternatives? A Systematic Review," *Annals of Internal Medicine* 157 (2012).

Taffy Brodesser-Akner, "Faith-Based Zucchini," *Pacific Standard,* June 6, 2013. www.psmag.com/health-and-behavior/safety-organic-food-genetically -modified-59279

Jon Hamilton, "Why You Shouldn't Panic About Pesticide in Produce," NPR .org, June 19, 2012. www.npr.org/blogs/thesalt/2012/06/19/155354070/why -you-shouldnt-panic-about-pesticide-in-produce

Tamar Haspel, "Is Organic Better for Your Health? A Look at Milk, Meat, Eggs, Produce and Fish," *Washington Post*, April 7, 2014.

Christie Wilcox, "Are Lower Pesticide Residues a Good Reason to Buy Organic? Probably Not," *Scientific American*, September 24, 2012.

Leah Zerbe, "2014 Dirty Dozen List: The Most Pesticide-Laden Produce You're Eating," *Rodale News,* April 29, 2014.

Fevers

Toby Bilanow, "The Benefits of Fever," *New York Times*, January 10, 2011.

Avery Hurt, "Benefits of Having a Fever," Parents.com, accessed September 1, 2014. www.parents.com/health/fever/fever-benefits/

Perri Klass, "Lifting a Veil of Fear to See a Few Benefits of Fever," *New York Times*, January 10, 2011.

Janice E. Sullivan and Henry C. Farrar, "Fever and Antipyretic Use in Children," *Pediatrics* 127, no. 3 (March 1, 2011): 580–587.

Allergies

Mike Martin, "The Mysterious Case of the Vanishing Genius," *Psychology To-day*, May 1, 2012.

Maggie Profet, "The Function of Allergy: Immunological Defense Against Tox- ins," *Quarterly Review of Biology* 66, no. 1 (March 1991): 23–62.

Melinda Wenner Moyer, "Are Allergies Trying to Protect Us from Ourselves?" PLOS.org, April 26, 2012. http://blogs.plos.org/bodypolitic/2012/04/26/are -allergies-trying-to-protect-us-from-ourselves/

BPAs

Jon Entine, "Bisphenol A (BPA) Found Not Harmful, Yet Again—So Why Did So Many Reporters and NGOs Botch Coverage, Yet Again?" *Forbes*, Octo- ber 31, 2012.

Jon Hamilton, "Maybe That BPA in Your Canned Food Isn't So Bad After All,"

NPR.com, February 26, 2014. www.npr.org/blogs/thesalt/2014/02/26/283030949/government-studies-suggest-bpa-exposure-from-food-isn-t-risky

David Ropeik, *How Risky Is It, Really? Why Our Fears Don't Always Match the Facts*, McGraw-Hill, 2012.

Justin Worland, "Why 'BPA-Free' May Be Meaningless" *Time*, April 15, 2015.

Katherine Zeratsky, "What Is BPA, and What Are the Concerns About BPA?" MayoClinic.com, May 21, 2013. www.mayoclinic.org/healthy-lifestyle/nutrition-and-healthy-eating/expert-answers/bpa/faq-20058331

Sunshine

Catharine Paddock, "Sun Exposure Benefits May Outweigh Risks Say Scientists," *Medical News Today*, May 8, 2013. www.medicalnewstoday.com/articles/260247.php

Catherine Shore-Lorenti et al., "Shining the Light on Sunshine: A Systematic Review of the Influence of Sun Exposure on Type 2 Diabetes Mellitus-Related Outcomes," *Clinical Endocrinology* 2014, doi: 10.1111/cen.12567.

Sadness

Joseph Forgas, "Don't Worry, Be Sad! On the Cognitive, Motivational, and Interpersonal Benefits of Negative Mood," *Association for Psychological Science* (SAGE Journals), 2013, doi: 10.1177/0963721412474458.

Daniel Kahneman, *Thinking, Fast and Slow,* Farrar, Straus and Giroux, 2011.

Bugs

Cayte Bosler, "To Save the World, Eat Bugs," *Atlantic*, February 25, 2014.

Michael Pollan, *The Omnivore's Dilemma: A Natural History of Four Meals*, Penguin, 2007.

Texas A&M AgriLife Communications, "Food Shortages Could Be Most Critical World Issue by Mid-century," ScienceDaily.com, April 17, 2014. www.sciencedaily.com/releases/2014/04/140417124704.htm

MORE FOOD
Steak

Kirsty Buchanan, "News to Sink Your Teeth into, Red Meat Is Good for You," *Express.co.uk*, June 30, 2013. www.express.co.uk/life-style/health/411327/News-to-sink-your-teeth-into-red-meat-is-good-for-you

Gary Taubes, *Why We Get Fat: And What to Do About It*, Anchor, 2011.

Nina Teicholz, *The Big Fat Surprise: Why Butter, Meat and Cheese Belong in a Healthy Diet*, Simon & Schuster, 2014.

Eggs

Nicholas Bakalar, "Eggs Regain Reputation," *New York Times*, January 28, 2013.

Tim Ferriss, *The 4-Hour Body: An Uncommon Guide to Rapid Fat-Loss, Incredible Sex, and Becoming Superhuman*, Harmony, 2010.

Kathleen Zelman, "Good Eggs: For Nutrition, They're Hard to Beat," WebMD.com, accessed October 2, 2014. www.webmd.com/diet/good-eggs-for-nutrition-theyre-hard-to-beat

Antibiotics in Red Meat

Michael Apley, "Consumers Hear Only Half the Story on Food-Borne Illness," *Beef*, March 25, 2014.

Associated Press, "Are Antibiotics in Meat Bad for Humans?" April 20, 2012, CBSNews.com, www.cbsnews.com/news/are-antibiotics-in-meat-bad-for-humans/

Dan Charles, "Are Farm Veterinarians Pushing Too Many Antibiotics?" NPR.com, November 1, 2013. www.npr.org/blogs/thesalt/2013/11/01/240278912/are-farm-veterinarians-pushing-too-many-antibiotics

MSG

Rachel Feltman, "No, MSG Isn't Bad for You," *Washington Post*, August 25, 2014.

Natasha Geiling, "It's the Umami, Stupid. Why the Truth About MSG Is So Easy to Swallow," *Smithsonian*. November 8, 2013.

U.S. Food and Drug Administration, "Questions and Answers on Monosodium glutamate (MSG)," FDA.gov, November 19, 2012. www.fda.gov/Food/IngredientsPackagingLabeling/FoodAdditivesIngredients/ucm328728.htm

Ice Cream

"Eating Ice Cream May Help Women to Conceive, But Low-Fat Dairy Foods May Increase Infertility Risk," *Medical News Today*, March 5, 2007. www.medicalnewstoday.com/articles/64192.php

Allison Knott, "Is FroYo Really Healthier Than Ice Cream?" *Boston Magazine*, August 20, 2013.

Holly McCord, *The Ice Cream Diet*, St. Martin's Press, 2002.

Carbs

Gary Taubes, *Why We Get Fat: And What to Do About It*, Anchor, 2011.

Junk Food

Tim Ferriss, *The 4-Hour Body: An Uncommon Guide to Rapid Fat-Loss, Incredible Sex, and Becoming Superhuman*, Harmony, 2010.

Aaron Gilbreath, "A Day Spent Eating Nothing but Dark Chocolate," *Men's Health*, October 2, 2014.

Courtney Hutchison, "Nutritionist Does Twinkie and Steak Diet, Loses Weight," ABCNews.com, September 20, 2010. http://abcnews.go.com/Health/Recipes/twinkie-diet-short-term-fix-long-term-problem/story?id=11756710

Angela Moore, "The Secret to a Long Life? Fast Food," *MarketWatch*, September 9, 2014. www.marketwatch.com/story/the-secret-to-a-long-life-fast-food-2014-09-08

FINAL THOUGHTS

Larry Copeland, "Life Expectancy in the USA Hits a Record High," *USA Today*, October 9, 2014.

Index

THE
BAD
NEWS
ABOUT WHAT'S GOOD FOR YOU

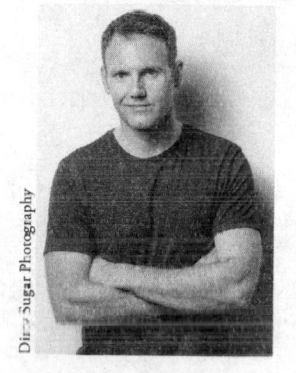

Jeff Wilser is a writer whose work has appeared in print or online in *New York* magazine, *GQ*, *Esquire*, *Mental Floss*, the *Los Angeles Times*, the *Chicago Tribune*, and *The Huffington Post*. In addition to writing about health, Wilser has covered a wide range of topics that includes books, monks, dating and relationships, business, man caves, sneak attacks of World War II, film, fashion (not that he's fashionable), and the out-of-control abuse of hashtags. (#Seriously.) His TV appearances span from BBC News to *The View*. He lives in Brooklyn, where he continues to personally research the medicinal benefits of whiskey, beer, and bacon. You can find him on Twitter at @JeffWilser.

THE
BAD
NEWS

ABOUT WHAT'S GOOD FOR YOU

JEFF WILSER

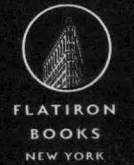

FLATIRON
BOOKS
NEW YORK

www.flatironbooks.com

Interior illustrations © David Curtis Studio
Interior design by Michelle McMillian
Cover design by Karen Horton
Cover illustrations © Shutterstock

The Library of Congress Cataloging-in-Publication Data is available upon request.

ISBN 978-1-250-06380-9 (hardcover)
ISBN 978-1-250-06381-6 (e-book)

Our books may be purchased in bulk for promotional, educational, or business use.
Please contact your local bookseller or the Macmillan Corporate and
Premium Sales Department at (800) 221-7945, extension 5442,
or by e-mail at MacmillanSpecialMarkets@macmillan.com.

First Edition: December 2015

10 9 8 7 6 5 4 3 2 1

To the health nuts: I'm sorry.
To the rest of us: You're welcome.

Contents

FITNESS   93
Standing Desks • Ball Chairs • Stretching • Diets •
Infomercial Fitness Products • Yoga • CrossFit •
Exercise

EVERYTHING ELSE   113
Marriage • Choice • News • College Degrees •
Height • Retirement • Moderation • Laughter

AUTHOR'S NOTE

This is not a how-to guide to health. Use it for informational purposes only. Consult with your doctor before making any changes. Read labels and warnings carefully, avoid extremes, and always listen to your body. (In other words, please don't swear off vegetables.)

Introduction

A while back I did a juice cleanse. Everything about it had the trappings of health: I "reset the system" and "purged my body of toxins." I did this for five days. Everything was gloriously *natural*. No pesticides, coffee, booze, bacon, eggs, or fat. No gluten. No evil GMOs. I plunked down $120 for a juicer, I bought sack after sack of organic fruit, and each morning, for nearly an hour, I liquefied a day's worth of carrots. Two things happened:

1. I doubled my grocery bill.
2. I felt like shit.

It turns out that your body needs things like protein, fat, and a little something the health experts call "food." Yes, a juice cleanse can help you temporarily lose weight, but that's just because you starve your body of calories. It's not complicated. (I did the same thing in my "junk cleanse" and it was far more enjoyable.) There's

no solid science behind a juice cleanse. It's counterproductive. It's a quick and easy way for us to *feel healthy* without addressing the underlying drivers of health.

My goal here isn't to take cheap shots at juicing. (We'll do that later.) There's a sneakier dynamic at play, and we'll see it echo throughout this section of the book: in our zealotry to be healthy, we can make choices that backfire. Especially if we're acting on a fad. And especially if its leading champions are Nicole Richie and Gwyneth Paltrow. We, as a culture, are easily seduced by panaceas. We want new, new, new! Maybe it's because the Age of Twitter feeds us new content every second of every hour. Just as there's an endless supply of tech news (better laptops! smartphones!), we're trained to crave the next big thing in health news. We seek "movements."

Yes, plenty of health food is actually healthy—I won't knock spinach—but much of what's framed as "healthy" is just a wolf in sheep's clothing. We have a Pavlovian response that associates "organic" with "healthy," but they make organic gummy bears and organic jelly beans. We drink Vitaminwater to be healthy, only to gulp down water that's spiked with sugar. Ditto for fruit juice. We gobble up frozen yogurt because it has yogurt in the name—and yogurt's healthy, right?—forgetting that *even in moderation* it's not much better than ice cream.

This goes beyond food and drink. New research suggests that much of what we think about fitness, medicine, education, and even brushing our teeth is outdated, unnecessary, or flat-out wrong. Most of us were taught to stretch before we go for a run or lift weights. Nope. Not only does static stretching have no benefit, it makes our muscles weaker. Multivitamins are a $40 billion industry, but in most mainstream studies, they do no better than a

placebo. Same for herbal supplements. Many of us feel guilty about sitting at the office all day, so we might try a stand-up desk or one of those iso-ball chairs, hoping to stay more active and burn more calories. Nope: the evidence says there's no health benefit, it ups the risk of injury, and when you sit on a bouncy-ball chair, you're 45 percent more likely to feel like a weirdo.

We'll explore the serious stuff like mammogram screenings, blood pressure drugs, and breast-feeding, and we'll also screw around a bit with the oddball downsides of laughter, retirement, and even height. (Being tall could be bad for you. George Costanza, you're welcome.)

But cheer up! Even though this is framed as "bad news" about what's good for you, as we'll see in the coming chapters, the bad news is actually good news. We bend over backwards to be healthy . . . even when it's not necessary. If we can identify where to cut corners without much downside, doesn't that make life simpler? If we're in good cardiovascular shape but we aren't the magazine version of skinny, maybe that's just as healthy—or even healthier. Instead of feeling sheepish that we don't get an annual physical, take comfort in the fact that, according to some doctors, they're a waste of your time.

Another reason why all this matters: sometimes the pursuit of the "most pure" can distract from the basics. *Eat in moderation, exercise in moderation.* So simple, so obvious, so true. Yet that headline won't fetch clicks. It won't carry a segment on a morning show. Instead we're exposed to new superfoods, new workouts, new diets. Let's say that we read some article entitled "1,000 Reasons to Eat More Avocados!" Now there's nothing inherently wrong with avocados. The danger, though, is when we buy our avocados, dump them in our large bowl of pasta, pat ourselves on the back,

and mentally check the health box . . . without fixing our underlying bad habits. Superfoods aren't a panacea.

We tend to fetishize food. We fetishize health. It's a status sym-
bol. Those in a certain demographic know that it's gauche to brag
about their BMWs, but it's perfectly acceptable, even encouraged,
to Instagram a $200 meal and hashtag #FarmToTable. There are
many solid reasons to eat local: to support honest farmers, to help
the environment, or maybe you just think it tastes better. (It often
does.) But is it actually *healthier*? The science, at best, is mixed.
This helps explain why there's a gap, at times, between the data and
our feelings.

This section of the book will strip away the fetish, peel off the
labels, and question how much of what's good for us actually lives
up to its hype.

Again, this is good news. Honest. If you've ever kicked yourself for not eating "clean enough," not running enough, or not buying enough kale, this is for you.

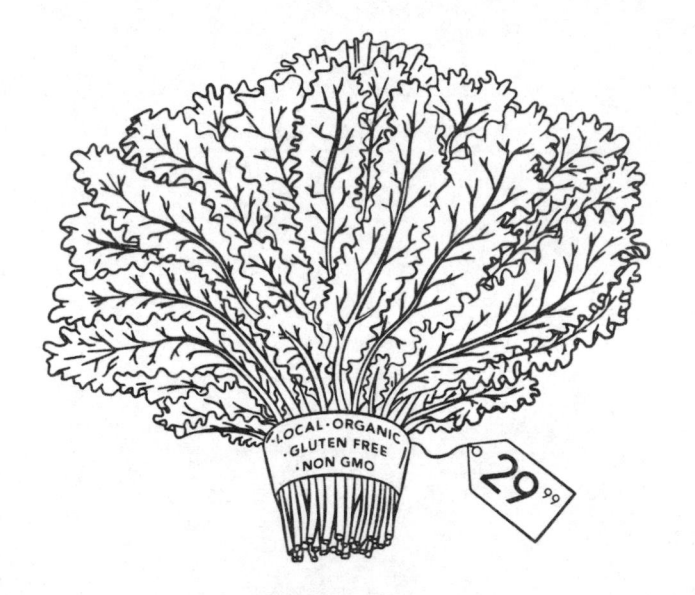

LOCAL·ORGANIC
·GLUTEN FREE
·NON GMO

29⁹⁹

FOOD

The only time to eat diet food is while you're waiting for the steak to cook. —Julia Child

Kale

Just a few signs that kale might be overrated:

- There's a National Kale Day. It's held the first Wednesday in October.
- The Kale-Heads are trying to convert you. The overlords at NationalKaleDay.org advise their minions to "Make your newbie their favorite food and 'sneak in' a little kale. Toss thinly sliced kale into noodle dishes, or chop kale in a food processor and add to meatloaf, turkey or lentil-based, or burger meat mixture." Let me repeat that. *They're sneaking kale into burgers.*
- We now live in a world with "kale chips" and "kale burrito shells."
- In Australia, a surge in demand caused a shortage of seeds, prompting Quartz.com to post "A Survival Guide for the Global Kale Crisis."
- *US Weekly* ran a splashy "Stars Who Love Kale" story that featured Jennifer Aniston, Gwyneth Paltrow (because of course), Heidi Klum, and Bette Midler. As Kevin Bacon says, "It's the age of kale. . . . A day without kale is like a day without sunshine."

But can too much kale actually kill you? Maybe. A mini kale backlash (or "anti-kalcism," as *The Observer*'s Drew Grant calls it) started with Jennifer Berman, a writer who was "into health food before it was cool" and juiced with kale every morning. "In the Whole Foods era, as I push my shopping cart down spacious aisles stocked with nonprocessed, gluten-free, non-G.M.O., heirloom, grass-fed, free-range and artisanal goods, I am pleased to know that I was ahead of my time," she writes in "Kale? Juicing? Trouble Ahead" for *The New York Times*. She was shocked to discover that kale should be avoided for women with hyperthyroidism, she learned that her juicing was bad for her teeth, and she closed the article by reaching for a Twinkie.

Any truth to this? Sort of. Kale is packed with goitrotgens, which, in whopping doses, could interfere with thyroid synthesis. But this would take roughly fifteen cups a day. For most people it's nothing to fear. The larger point is that, yes, kale is healthy, but so are almost all vegetables. It's not a miracle food. There are no miracle foods. We like shortcuts in health, so we think that if we *just change one thing*—like incorporating kale—suddenly we'll drop weight and boost our energy and finally read that growing stack of *New Yorkers*. Kale gives us hope. "Kale is the 'food of the moment,' following in the footsteps of blueberries, acai berries, mango, etc. It is a nutrient-dense green veggie, but no more so than other green veggies," Dr. Katherine Beals, a nutrition expert at the University of Utah, tells me. And for most people, there's nothing to worry about as "the thyroid thing is crap."

So eat your kale, like all things, in moderation. Scientists have proven that too much kale, especially if you live in Brooklyn, might cause death from an overdose of smugness.

"Low Fat"

There's only one thing I hate more than lying: skim milk,
which is water that's lying about being milk.

—Ron Swanson

Here's the fundamental problem: fat tastes good. So when a company designs a food that's "fat-free," "low-fat," or "reduced-fat," they run the risk that it will taste like bark. Studies have shown that bark doesn't sell. Solution: load the bastard up with sugar. Since sugar, technically, isn't a fat, they can slap on a cheery "fat-free!" label and give us the illusion that we're being healthy.

It's one hell of a con. The makers of low-fat products "remove a little of the fat and its calories, but then replace it with carbohydrates. In the case of low-fat yogurt, for instance, they replace much of the fat removed with high-fructose corn syrup," notes Gary Taubes, who deserves much of the credit for exposing the true cost of this trade-off. "We think we're eating a heart-healthy, low-fat snack that will lead to weight loss. Instead, we get fatter because of the added carbohydrates and fructose."

Things that are "low-fat" or "fat-free":

- Frosted Flakes
- Skittles
- Coke
- Fat-free cookies
- Cocaine
- Broccoli

Of course there's nothing wrong with broccoli. It's on the list to clarify that by "low fat," I don't mean every single food that's absent of fat, but rather foods that normally contain fat (like butter), but have then been chemically altered to swap the fat with sugar, flour, or Flavorizer #3,407. Almost all nutritionists seem to agree on this: even in the holy wars of low fat versus low carb, the experts agree that plants and vegetables are an unqualified good, and that highly processed "low-fat" foods are misleading at best, poison at worst.

The low-fat cookie, in a sense, is an allegory for an overall low-fat diet. When you give up fat you have to replace it with *something*. If you're so iron-willed that you can replace the fat with carrots, good on you. For most people, though, the trade-off is for refined carbohydrates. I'm one of the suckers. For years, when I saw two competing brands in the grocery store, one with 18 grams of fat and one labeled fat-free, I'd grab the fat-free without blinking. I bought low-fat cereal. Fat-free milk. This goes back to the iconic Food Pyramid and what we were taught in third grade. *Fat makes us fat.* The homonym is a powerful thing.

But what about the studies that show that low-fat diets work? It just seems like common sense. If we expunge ice cream and butter from our diet, that's gotta help, right?

The pro-fat camp has two responses. The first: Yes, there might be studies showing that a low-fat diet can help you lose weight, but other studies show that low-carb, high-fat diets have done even better.

The second response: Even when caloric-restricted diets are billed as low-fat, when they work, they have the unintended consequence of *also reducing the overall carb intake*—a good thing. When we cut fatty foods like ice cream and donuts, we're also

cutting carbs and sugar. Ironically, this is the mirror image of the argument that the low-fat camp makes when low-carb, high-fat diets work: they say that when you cut carbs, you're also slashing the overall calories.

Whether you follow the Taubes and Teicholz wing of nutrition—*eat fat, avoid cheap carbs*—or the Katz model of *whole foods and sensible choices,* there's not much reason to eat "reduced-fat" foods. So if it's a choice between a sugary substitute and the fatty real thing, go with the fat. Besides, you already know what no study can quantify: it just tastes better.

> The technical differences between the labels, as per *WebMD*:
>
> **"Fat-free":** Less than 0.5 gram of fat per serving
>
> **"Low-fat":** Less than 3 grams of fat per serving
>
> **"Reduced-fat":** Less than 25 percent the fat of the regular versions
>
> **"Light":** Either ⅓ fewer calories or 50 percent less fat

Breakfast

Your grandma said the same thing as my grandma, who said the same thing as every doctor and health expert on the planet: breakfast is the most important meal of the day. The logic seems bulletproof: When we eat early in the day, we kick-start our metabolism, replenish energy, and curb hunger pangs.

Or maybe not. Recent studies have dared to challenge this

bedrock of nutrition, testing whether, for people who are trying to lose weight, it's more effective to eat or skip breakfast. At the University of Alabama, researchers took three hundred volunteers (who were trying to diet) and split them into three groups:

Group 1: They were told to *eat breakfast*, and given a pamphlet on a good diet.

Group 2: They were told to *skip breakfast*, and given a pamphlet on a good diet.

Group 3: They were given a pamphlet on a good diet. (They could *eat or skip* as they preferred.)

They did this for about four months. And as the lead researcher, Dr. David Allison, told me, "There was no difference in weight loss. Our study suggests that—at least in adults who want to lose weight—when choosing between eating breakfast every day and skipping breakfast every day, it doesn't matter."

How is this possible? If we miss breakfast, doesn't our body slip into "starvation mode," slow the metabolism, and then, at noon, get ambushed by a roast beef sandwich? As Allison explains it to me, the traditional rationale for why it's important to eat breakfast is that, if you skip it, you'll be so hungry that at lunchtime, you'll devour *even more calories* than you skipped at breakfast. Yet that's not what happened. Maybe the Breakfast Skippers ate a bit more at lunch, but not enough to tip the scales.

But what about that old chestnut, "Eat breakfast like a king, lunch like a prince, and dinner like a pauper"? At least one study suggests that this, too, might still have legs. A 2013 experiment from Tel Aviv University split fifty overweight women into two

groups. Both groups were instructed to go on a diet of 1,400 calories a day. The only difference? The *timing* of those calories.

> *Group 1:* 1,400 calories a day, with a 200-calorie breakfast,
> 500-calorie lunch, 700-calorie dinner. While the calorie
> count is puny, this is a rough approximation of our typi-
> cal eating habits—toast for breakfast, sandwich for lunch,
> platter of food for dinner.
>
> *Group 2:* 1,400 calories a day, but with the meals reversed:
> 700-calorie breakfast, 500-calorie lunch, 200-calorie
> dinner.

Group 1, the large dinner group (the more traditional model),
lost 8 pounds. But the people who ate breakfast like kings lost *19
pounds*. They also showed improvement in their blood profile, with
lower levels of insulin and glucose. "Metabolism is impacted by
the body's circadian rhythm, the biological process that the body
follows over a 24-hour cycle. So the time of day we eat can have a
big impact on the way our bodies process food," said lead researcher
Dr. Daniela Jakubowicz.

How are both of these studies compatible? This is just my own
hypothesis, but in the second study (eat breakfast like a king),
the *total number of calories* was held constant, and when you do
this, they found it's better to front-load your calories in the morning. The study of Breakfast Skippers does *not* hold the calories
constant, so it's likely that when people ate breakfast, those calories bump the daily total higher.

Conclusion? Maybe it's case-by-case. As a sample size of one,
when I wake up in the morning, I need to eat something ASAP or

my blood sugar plummets and I scowl at puppies. I also have friends who never get hungry until lunch, and they bristle at people (like me) who tell them *you need to eat breakfast! Be healthy!* I will continue to eat breakfast, but maybe my breakfast-skipping buddy—who's in great shape and feels fine each morning—should no longer be harassed.

Predictably, there were several objections to this contrarian study, including:

- It was only conducted for four months; maybe if these people had been tracked for five years, it'd be a different story?
- They weren't told *what to eat* for breakfast; it's possible that if they were forced to eat a certain type of food, it'd be a different story.
- The experiment didn't study children, so we shouldn't extrapolate too much and issue guidelines for kid-raising.

As Allison tells me, "My reply to all of these limitations is . . . I agree. All of those are good points, and that's for future research." But he also points out that of the limited peer-review studies out there, *none* show that skipping breakfast has a negative effect. The evidence is consistent.

Soy

Soy will cause brain damage, and you should stop eating and drinking it immediately and start eating steak and drinking beer.

Sigh. Of course that's not true. As a meat eater who grew up in Texas, an evil little part of me would be delighted to take some

cheap shots at soy, cherry-picking the studies that suggest that soy might cause allergies or kidney disease. There's certainly plenty of fodder; when you do a search for "soy" in the research database PubMed, you get 13,557 results. People seem fascinated with trying to prove that it either lengthens our lives or causes breast cancer. This entire book could be on soy. I'll save both of us some time: the health community has largely given soy a thumbs-up. I love this curt reply from nutritionist Katherine Beals, when I asked her about soy. "It is a high-protein plant source. It will neither cure menopausal symptoms nor cause cancer in normal amounts." (So if you want to get technical, I suppose this is not really Bad News about soy but the Good News about the Bad News about soy.)

Frozen Yogurt

In the late 1980s, when frozen yogurt first became a thing, TCBY was originally known as "This Can't Be Yogurt!" Once we got used to the concept, TCBY realized that we're not a bunch of idiots—we get it—so they tweaked the acronym to "The Country's Best Yogurt." Since then, fro-yo has yo-yoed from strip-mall kitsch to health food staple to artisanal wonder; we now live in a world with Pinkberry, Red Mango, Twist, Yogurt Crazy, and Forever Yogurt. The Pretension Award goes to my local Brooklyn frozen yogurt shop, which simply calls itself *Culture*. (Also, free business idea—frozen yogurt marketed to men: BroYo.)

So what's so bad about fro-yo?

Short version: the problem isn't that it's *terrible,* and it's not bad for you in the way that, say, Ding-Dongs are bad for you, but it's a dessert that tries to pretend it's not a dessert. It's a fraud. It gives

the illusion of health. It gives us false confidence that we can pour the vanilla yogurt all the way to the top of the cup, higher, higher, just a little higher, and then drizzle it with caramel.

Fro-yo's main selling point: it's fat-free. But like most fat-free foods that aren't disgusting, to secure that coveted fat-free status, it makes the Faustian deal of loading up with sugar. Let's look at Pinkberry. (I'm using Pinkberry as an example, but you'll see the same sort of thing with most fro-yo companies.)

Each serving has 21 grams of sugar, and the serving size is "half a cup." But who only eats a half-cup of yogurt? It's worth looking closer. According to Pinkberry's website, this is how the sizes break down:

Mini: 0.9 servings
Small 1.4 servings
Medium 2.3
Large 3.7
Take Home 7.1

Even the damn Small is still 1.4 servings. I'm ashamed to admit that I usually order a Large when I visit Pinkberry (I'm also ashamed to admit that I've stepped inside a Pinkberry), but for the people with more willpower than me, let's look at a Medium. Medium should be average, right? A responsible portion of food? Pinkberry's Medium has 2.3 servings.

This means that for a Medium serving of Pinkberry fro-yo—which is billed as fat-free and therefore healthy, and since it's Medium, it feels like moderation—yo're getting 48 grams of sugar. And that's not even counting the toppings.

Alternatives to frozen yogurt that have less than 48 grams of sugar:

- 2 Hershey's bars
- 2 Almond Joys
- 2 Snickers
- 1 Milky Way
- A pack of Skittles
- A pack of Starburst
- A pack of Sour Patch Kids
- 2 packs of Jolly Rancher hard candies
- 2 packs of Twizzlers
- A pack of M&M's
- 22 Hershey's Kisses
- 2 packs of ROLOs
- 2 packs of Milk Duds
- 3 packets of Fun Dip. *Fun Dip.*

So will you die if you eat the occasional frozen yogurt? No. And I will continue to shame myself at Pinkberry. But you could make an argument that when you order ice cream, at least *you know it's dangerous,* and you will therefore, hopefully, choose your portion accordingly. A half-cup of ice cream versus a half-cup of fro-yo? Trick question. No one thinks that way. In reality, the calculus is usually a half-cup of ice cream versus two cups of fro-yo . . . and in that case you might as well savor the ice cream.

Maybe TCBY had it right all along. In some ways this can't be yogurt.

Fish

One week: Fish is good! The next week: Fish is bad! Fish has healthy fatty acids! Fish is poisoned with mercury!

So which is it? A source of lean protein, or something that might kill us?

By now you can guess the answer: both. Trade-offs exist. We've known about the threat of mercury poisoning since the 1950s, when, in Japan, a petrochemical company kinda-sorta dumped twenty-seven tons of something called methylmercury into the water. Oops! The fish absorbed the water. The people ate the fish. Nine hundred people died. Others were paralyzed, had seizures, and went blind. Babies were born with defects. It was something of a bad scene.

The good news—well, not for them, but for us—is that the Japan catastrophe was caused by a once-in-a-lifetime amount of mercury. Since then, the levels have plummeted. Study after study has shown that yes, there can be traces of mercury in fish, just as there are tiny traces of chemicals in almost everything we eat, but the levels are so low that they do not pose a material risk.*

Well . . . not *all* studies have shown that fish are harmless. In 2012, a report from the Biodiversity Research Institute suggested that "Threats from mercury are greater at lower levels than we have thought in the past," according to David Evers, the executive director of BRI. "The more we look at mercury, the more toxic it is."

---

*This doesn't mean the issue should be ignored. It's the very threat of mercury poisoning—and the looming public outrage—that led to stricter regulation of pollution. Watchdogs matter.

Others added to the chorus. "These are not trivial effects, these are significant effects," said Dr. Edward Groth, one of the researchers and an adviser to the World Health Organization. "There does appear to be evidence now, fairly persuasive evidence, that adverse effects occur from normal amounts of seafood consumption."

But other studies have drawn different conclusions, and on balance, for most people, health experts generally agree that the good almost certainly outweighs the bad. "Fish is an excellent source of omega-3 fatty acids and is the only natural source of the DHA and EPA. Yes, certain fish have a high mercury content and should, thus, be consumed sparingly," Dr. Beals tells me. "If you are concerned about mercury levels of fish, you can check the Environmental Protection Agency's Web site for a list of fish that have high and low mercury contents. Avoid those with high mercury levels, or consume them infrequently."

Narrowly focusing on the tiny risk of mercury poisoning might miss the big picture. It's similar to what risk expert David Ropeik called the "perception gap" that we saw with BPAs. Just as we'll see with salad, you're going to have to swap the fish for *something*, and that something will probably be worse for you. And fish brings so much to the table. "Oily fish like salmon, mackerel, bluefish, herring and sardines are rich in omega-3 fatty acids. These are polyunsaturated fatty acids that may protect against heart attacks and stroke, help control blood clotting and build cell membranes in the brain. They are also important to an infant's visual and neurological development," writes veteran food columnist Jane Brody in a piece called, well, "Lots of Reasons to Eat Fish." She echoes what other studies suggest—that the tiny, tiny risk of fetal mercury poisoning is outweighed by the benefits of fetal brain development. "Omega-3s may also help ameliorate a variety of conditions, such

as cancer, depression, inflammatory bowel disease, and autoimmune disorders like lupus and rheumatoid arthritis."*

Oh, and it's correlated with longer life spans, too. A 2013 study, led by Dr. Dariush Mozaffarian of Harvard, showed that fish-eaters tended to live 2.2 years longer than non-fish-eaters. The risk of heart disease was slashed by 35 percent. "Although eating fish has long been considered part of a healthy diet, few studies have assessed blood omega-3 levels and total deaths in older adults. Our findings support the importance of adequate blood omega-3 levels for cardiovascular health, and suggest that later in life these benefits could actually extend the years of remaining life," said Mozaffarian.

In response to questionable studies about the threat of mercury, an exasperated National Fisheries Institute wrote an open letter to journalists on "Errors and Distortions in News Coverage," pointing out specific news stories that, in their view, told only one very small part of the story, failing to put the benefits of fish in larger context. As far as nutritional debates go, it's juicy stuff. They blast various writers from *Vogue* to the AP to the *Chicago Tribune*, noting that, in each example, the paper ultimately issued a correction. Example: *Vogue* ran a piece called "Mercury Rising," and in response, the National Fisheries Institute charges, "[the writer] failed to mention the new, landmark FDA draft report on fish consumption that reported cognitive benefits for 99.9 percent of babies and young children, as well as its role in preventing 50,000 deaths a year from heart disease and stroke. Also ignored: years of

---

*Eating tuna while pregnant remains especially controversial. The FDA suggests 8 to 12 ounces a week, but an October 2014 analysis from Consumer Reports recommends a policy of Zero Tolerance. Talk to your doctor.

positive studies and reports on the benefits of increased fish consumption by *The Lancet*, the *Journal of the American Medical Association* and the Institute of Medicine."

Fish isn't free of risk. But *nothing* is free of risk. Consume accordingly.

Smoothies

See: Frozen Yogurt.

Quick anecdote that happened while I was writing this chapter: On a road trip with some friends, we hit a McDonald's drive-through. Two of us ordered ice-cream cones. I could tell the third friend wanted ice cream, but he was trying to be healthy, so he said, "I'll have a smoothie." He ordered a medium.

   Ice-cream cone: 170 calories, 27 grams of carbs, 20 grams
      of sugar
   Smoothie: 250 calories, 58 grams of carbs, 54 grams of sugar

Nuts

Every few weeks, you'll see an article called something like "7 Reasons to Eat More Nuts!" or "Nuts About Nuts!" and these articles, which show many photos of skinny people smiling, are bound to use phrases like:

   "Nutritional powerhouses!"
   "Super-food!"
   "Heart-friendly!"

"Antiaging wonders!"

"Brain-boosting!"

That's not necessarily wrong. The experts all seem to agree that, when consumed in moderation—allergies aside—nuts are the shit. So what's the rub? More than most other foods, the "in moderation" disclaimer is a crucial one.

Tim Ferriss found that while *in theory* it's fine to eat a few, in practice, this is just bad policy. "There are certain foods that, while technically fine to eat . . . are prone to portion abuse. I call these 'domino foods,' as eating one portion often creates a domino effect of oversnacking," he recommends in *The 4 Hour Body*. "My fat-loss has plateaued three times due to almonds, which are easy to consume by the handful and simple to excuse as nutritious. Unfortunately, they also contain 824 calories per cup, 146 calories more than a Whopper from Burger King (678 kilocalories). A few almonds is just fine (5–10), but no one eats just a few almonds."

Salad

Tony Soprano: I think it's time for you to start to seriously consider salads.

Bobby Baccalieri: What do you mean?

Tony Soprano: What do I mean? I mean get off my car before you flip it over, you fat fuck!

Salads. Even one of our nation's top nutritionists, Tony Soprano, knows that the key to health is to eat more salad. He has a

point. The health industry is splintered on issues like fat versus carbs, but almost everyone agrees on this one thing: leafy greens are good. They give us fiber and they help us feel full. As Michael Pollan famously said in what has to be the glummest advice in history, "Eat food. Not too much. Mostly plants."

So what's the rub? If I wanted to sensationalize things, I'd push a 2013 report from the CDC that found that leafy vegetables— lettuce, spinach, and our darling kale—are the top causes of food poisoning.* The authors of the study were quick to point out that people should continue to eat their greens. They urged us to rinse and wash vegetables.

The study makes for a provocative headline. And it neatly fits the cheeky premise of this book, so it's tempting to close this entry and call it a day.

But "salad causes food poisoning, therefore salad is unhealthy" is the wrong takeaway. If we avoid spinach on the basis of this logic, we again fall into that classic trap of health studies: blurring the relative risks with the absolute risks. Yes, perhaps it's true that in the cases where the CDC observed food poisoning, leafy greens made up a high percentage. It's also true that one in six Americans have food poisoning each year.

Your *absolute* risk of contracting food poisoning from leafy vegetables isn't that high, and it's only a smidge higher than if you had a diet with zero leafy vegetables. As a quick hypothetical, let's imagine you see this scary headline, "Leafy Greens: Leading Cause

---

* It used to be beef, but after the industry adopted tighter safety standards, red meat tumbled down the list. Despite all the hysteria about mad cow disease, beef is now responsible for less than 4 percent of deaths from food poisoning.

of Food Poisoning," and then you say to yourself, screw that, I'm never eating another bite of lettuce.

The problem is that leafy greens only account for 22 percent of all the cases of food poisoning—yes, it's a plurality, but it's nowhere near a majority. Since you will continue to eat food, you'd still be at risk for the other 78 percent, which includes dairy, poultry, meat, etc.

So, the simplified math:

Since one in six people get food poisoning each year—again, the math is simplified and it avoids demographic skews, your age, diet, etc.—your odds are basically one in six to begin with, if you were eating leafy greens. So each year you have a 16.7 percent chance of food poisoning (16.7 percent: 1 divided by 6). If you cut leafy greens from your diet, you'd remove 22 percent of that risk—which lowers your absolute risk of food poisoning from 16.7 percent to 13 percent (16.7 percent multiplied by 78 percent = 13 percent).

Already the headline is far less shocking: "Leafy Greens Might Cause Modest Risk in Food Poisoning, from 13 percent to 17 percent." But let's be honest. Food poisoning *itself* isn't (usually) that serious a health risk. Yes, it's profoundly unpleasant, and it's an excellent way to ruin your afternoon, but it's not really a legit *health risk* unless you're hospitalized. The CDC gives us those figures, too. Each year there are 128,000 hospitalizations due to food poisonings. As we have a population of 319 million, that means that the odds of hospitalization due to food poisoning is 0.04 percent. If we remove leafy greens from our diet, then we still have a 78 percent of the overall risk, which trims the number to . . . drumroll, please . . . 0.03 percent. (0.04 percent multiplied by 78 percent = 0.03 percent.)

If we round to the nearest tenth decimal point, which is custom:

If you eat leafy greens, odds of hospitalization from food
poisoning: 0.0 percent
If you do *not* eat leafy greens, odds of hospitalization from
food poisoning: 0.0 percent

It's a rounding error. And it's certainly not a reason to skip salad. In the dozen or so articles I read about this study when it came out, nowhere did I see this math. We rarely talk about absolute risk. Instead, a more typical analysis was the opening line from this story at CBS: "Eating your greens might be hazardous to your health."

Our analysis isn't yet complete. Hypothetically, if you refuse to eat leafy vegetables, you might have reduced your odds of food

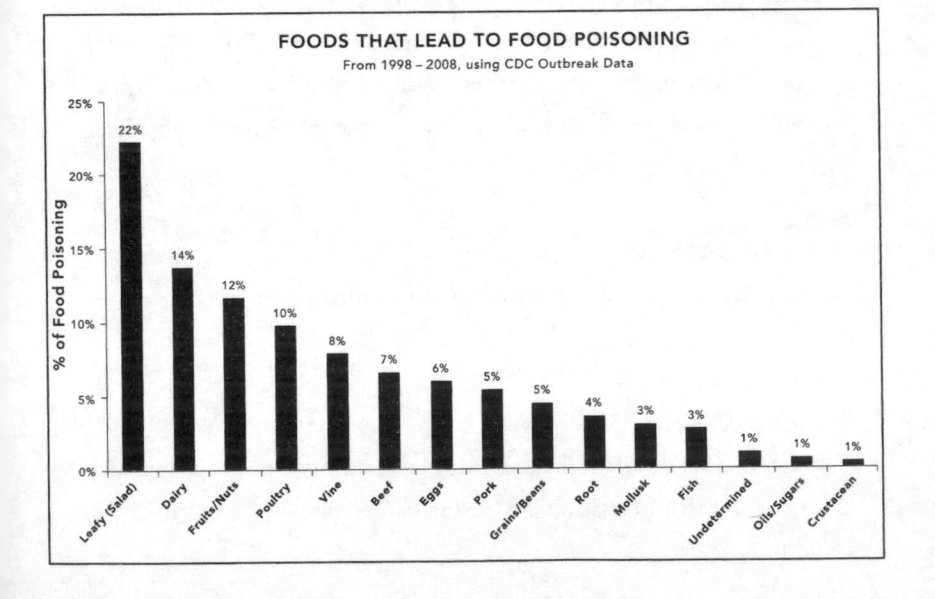

FOODS THAT LEAD TO FOOD POISONING
From 1998 – 2008, using CDC Outbreak Data

poisoning hospitalization from 0.04 percent to 0.03 percent, but that's only the tiniest slice of your overall health risk. If you cut lettuce from your diet, something else has surely taken its place. More pasta, more nuts, more Pop-Tarts? Whatever it is, your odds of *something else bad* have gone up. If you replaced the lettuce with more sugar or refined carbs, for example, you just spiked your risk of diabetes.

The point isn't to extol the virtues of lettuce—you don't need me for that. Salad has its guardians. The point is that, back to the concept of trade-offs, even the best of foods can have *something* wrong with them, but if we focus too much on any one study—especially if we read no further than the headline in our Twitter feed—it might nudge us from healthy behavior. This same logic is why maybe we shouldn't freak out over BPA, pesticides, or antibiotics in red meat.

Salad does have one legit problem: a salad is rarely just a salad. It can be a delivery mechanism for a platter of sugar and carbs. Salads are often loaded with breaded chicken, dried fruits, and dressing that's laced with sugar. *Men's Health* provides a handy roundup of "20 Salads Worse than a Whopper," including:

Jack in the Box
Crispy Chicken Club Salad with Croutons and
Ranch Dressing: **873 calories**

El Pollo Loco
Chicken Tostada Salad with Light Creamy
Cilantro Dressing: **910 calories**

Quizno's
Chicken Caesar Flatbread Salad (with bread):
   920 calories

California Pizza Kitchen
Field Greens Salad with Gorgonzola Cheese:
   1,098 calories

Cosi
Cobb Salad: **708 calories**

So there's nothing wrong with a salad . . . assuming it's an honest-to-god salad and not a few scraps of lettuce that camouflage a Big Mac. To paraphrase the NRA, *salads don't kill, toppings do.**

Margarine

Butter is delicious. Butter is honest. Butter has been used for centuries.

Margarine, on the other hand, is a synthetic Frankenfood that was spawned from our fear of saturated fats. It's a recent invention. Margarine was glorified as the "healthy alternative" to butter. We thought it made us skinnier. We thought it lowered our cholesterol.

---

* This is neither an endorsement nor a swipe at the NRA. I'm making enough enemies in this book with the health stuff; I'll save my thoughts on gun control for the sequel.

Nope. "For years, margarine was promoted as a heart-healthy alternative to butter. Since margarine was made from unsaturated vegetable oils, most people assumed it would be better for long-term health than butter, which was known to contain a lot of cholesterol and saturated fat. That assumption turned out to be wrong," states the Harvard School of Public Health. "Research showed that some forms of margarine—specifically the hard-stick margarines—were worse for the heart than butter." Or as Rochelle Bilow, a friend and food writer for *Bon Appétit*, tells me, "Butter is kind of like sex (stay with me here): It's great even when it's mediocre. But *good* butter? The stuff made from cows that ate lush pasture and grazed freely outside? That's arguably the world's most perfect food. It's grassy, it's sweet, and just the right amount of funky."

Fruit

This is controversial. Most health experts agree that fruit is good. They point out that fruit is packed with fiber, vitamins, and nutrients. All of this is true.

But it's also true that fruit is full of sugar. Lots of it.

According to the American Heart Association, we should cap our daily sugar intake between 26 grams (for women) and 36 grams (for men). One orange has 23 grams of sugar.

But, but, but . . . how can this be? Fruits are one of the good guys, right? Ever since I was a little kid, I've been told to eat "more fruits and vegetables." And it's funny how those two words always travel in tandem—fruits and vegetables.

Maybe this is part of the problem. "Lumping together 'fruits

and vegetables' . . . that was just crazy," Teicholz tells me. "It's such a crazy thing to do. Fruits are very high in sugar. They're the favored snacks by all schools, but they're not as good for you as you'd think."

This doesn't mean we should swear off apples and strawberries. But to Teicholz's point, our conflation of "fruits and vegetables" means that we tend to suck them down with impunity, giving a banana the same moral force as broccoli. A more accurate bundling might be "fruits and sweets" or "fruits and cakes." It's true that bananas have fiber, just as it's true that cheesecake has calcium. (True, that's not a fair comparison. It's not really fair to bananas or, frankly, to cheesecake.)

But consider. The average banana has 13 grams of sugar. A slice of cheesecake has 27. This has consequences. As a midmorning snack, for example, most of us aren't reaching for a wedge of cheese-cake. Bananas? Different story. I'll snack on one in the morning and another in the afternoon, congratulating myself on my healthy choices—after all I'm eating *fruits and vegetables*.

Sugar is sugar. And the nutrition industry is beginning to pivot, with more and more nutritionists declaring that sugar, not fat, is Public Enemy number one. In 2014, the World Health Organization *cut in half* the recommended daily sugar intake, from 10 percent of calories to 5 percent.

It's easy to train our anger at Coke and Skittles, and yes, it's almost certainly true that cheesecake sugar is worse than banana sugar. However . . . "As nutritionists and public-health authorities have become increasingly desperate in their attempts to rein in the obesity epidemic, they've also become increasingly strident in their suggestions that we eat copious fruit along with green vegetables. Maybe so," writes Gary Taubes, whose "Is Sugar Toxic?" manifesto

helped shape the debate. "But if we're predisposed to put on fat, it's a good bet that most fruit will make the problem worse, not better." Taubes is not saying that all of us should stop eating fruit. But if someone's obese? Think twice about loading up on apples.

That said, and I can't stress this enough, most experts—including those in the anti-sugar crowd—encourage eating fruit in moderation. Dr. Katz was clearly exasperated at having to *defend* the consumption of fruit, writing, "Despite the idea that fructose is toxic, it IS still okay to eat whole, fresh fruits. Geez!" He also says, "You find me the person who can legitimately blame their obesity or diabetes on apples or carrots, and I will give up my day job and become a hula dancer!"

Organic Food

There are plenty of reasons to buy organic. You might find that it tastes better. You might argue that it's better for the environment. You might insist that when it comes to the treatment of, say, chickens, organic is more humane.*

But is it actually *healthier?* The science, once again, is mixed.

The organic food industry is massive. With over $35 billion in annual revenue, it's no longer the feel-good underdog. Three out of four grocery stores carry organic food, according to the USDA. "Organic" is a word that people conflate with "healthy"—this is how we justify the price premium.

In 2012, this industry wasn't too pleased about a report from

---

* "Treatment," of course, is a euphemism for "slaughter."

Stanford, where a meta-analysis of over two hundred studies, led by Dr. Dena Bravata, found that after crunching all the numbers and weighing all the relevant experiments, the data "lacks strong evidence that organic foods are significantly more nutritious than conventional foods." When it came to nutrition and vitamins, organic and conventional were a toss-up. "I was absolutely surprised," said Bravata. "There are many reasons why someone might choose organic foods over conventional foods," she said, but for nutritional value, "there isn't much difference." Another coauthor said, "Some believe that organic food is always healthier and more nutritious. We were a little surprised that we didn't find that." After Stanford threw down this gauntlet, two predictable things happened:

1. The media went nuts, running headlines like AP's: "Organic Food Is Not Healthier than Conventional Produce: Study."
2. The Organic Empire strikes back, pointing out the study's fine print. The Stanford study *also* concluded that organic foods did have a lower pesticide level than conventional foods.

Critics of the study said that we don't eat organic food to consume more vitamin B, we do it to have cleaner food. "The study was like declaring guns no more dangerous than baseball bats when it comes to blunt-object head injuries. It was the equivalent of comparing milk and Elmer's glue on the basis of whiteness. It did, in short, miss the point," writes Mark Bittman. "How can something that reduces your exposure to pesticides and antibiotic-resistant bacteria not be 'more nutritious' than food that doesn't?"

It's a fair question. And the answer really depends on your risk tolerance, and whether you think that the level of pesticides in conventional food—which, admittedly, is higher than in organic—is high enough to pose a material risk. Plenty of data says it's not. As Christie Wilcox writes in *Scientific American*, "Yes, conventional foods have more synthetic pesticide residues than organic ones, on average. And yes, pesticides are dangerous chemicals. But does the science support paying significantly more for organic foods just to avoid synthetic pesticides? No." The dosage isn't high enough to pose an absolute risk.

I would argue that there's a sneakier problem with organic foods: they're yet one more illusion that we're being healthy. Sometimes we are and sometimes we're not. "We don't have definite evidence that eating organic *improves* human health," Dr. Katz tells me, adding that he personally recommends buying organic for the "dirty dozen," just in case. "But some people get so carried away with the Organic Halo Effect, they think it doesn't matter what the food is. Given the choice between non-organic broccoli and organic gummy bears, I'd go with the non-organic broccoli."*

---

*There are differences on a case-by-case basis; some people find that their bodies react better to organic food. Some people have allergies. It's entirely possible that this type of nuance wouldn't be caught in a massive study. If you find that organic tastes better, sits with you better, or simply feels like a higher quality of food, that's a legit reason to buy organic. No study has ever shown that HDTV televisions are better for our health than old Standard Definition televisions, but there's no way I'm going back. Preferences matter.

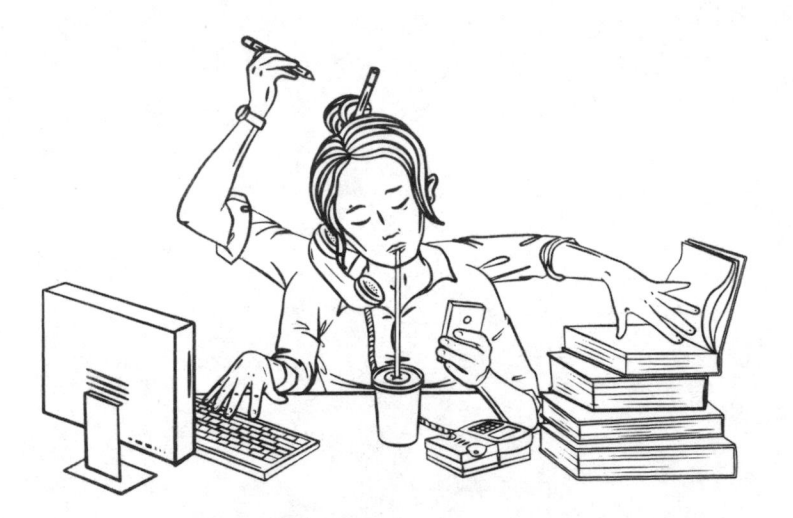

HABITS

Remember how back in high school, some of the "gunners"—
the ones who never relaxed, studied on Saturday night,
and had nightmares about getting a B+—were the most
miserable kids in the school? There's something to this.
Sometimes healthy habits *can* backfire, just like healthy
diets.

Homework

If you're under the age of eighteen, put this down right now or your parents will sue me.

I mean it.

Okay. So here's the deal. Study after study has shown that our kids are burdened with too much homework. It's causing stress, it's triggering burnout, it's exhausting the parents, and, most important, it could be self-defeating.

"Our findings on the effects of homework challenge the traditional assumption that homework is inherently good," explains Stanford researcher Denise Pope, who, in 2014, studied four thousand students in upper-middle-class California suburbs, finding that while they might be notching A's, it's not translating into learning or engagement.

This doesn't mean that all homework is evil. Pope isn't some radical who wants to see it banished. "Homework can be great for you if it's meaningful, purposeful, and developmentally appropriate," she tells me.

"So where do we draw the line?"

That line might be closer to zero than you'd think. A proper analysis of the education system is just a tad outside the scope of the book, but let's quickly consider the work of Harris Cooper, an education guru who pored through the results of 170 different studies of homework. When the dust settled, as Pope says, "There's

almost zero correlation between homework and academic success at the elementary school level. In the middle school there's a *slight* correlation, but it drops off at ninety minutes a night. And at high school there's a strong correlation, but it drops off at two hours."

So for a lazy sophomore who spends all his time killing zombies on the Xbox, yes, he should get his ass off the couch and hit the bio-chem. "But we've got kids doing four or five hours a night," says Pope, and it's counterproductive.

About fifteen years ago, Pope shadowed five high school students for an entire school year. "I found some high-achieving kids who were great kids, but they were stressed out, completely disengaged, even though they had high GPAs. They were playing the game and not really learning for learning's sake." This spawned her book *Doing School: How We Are Creating a Generation of Stressed-Out, Materialistic, and Miseducated Students*, and helped launch Challenge Success, which pushes for a rethinking of how we evaluate our students.

"We think of homework as a 'take your medicine because it's good for you,'" she says, "But it's taking away from their *downtime* and child playtime. It's causing stress on the families. I hear parents tell me all the time, 'When I'm helping my kid for two hours with homework, I can't cook dinner or get laundry done.'"

Studies around the globe have found similar results. A psychologist at Sydney University, Richard Walker, found that when looking across countries, there *is*, in fact, a correlation between homework and the scores of standardized tests . . . but the correlation is inverse. Nations that spend the most time on homework tend to perform the worst, and vice versa. Take Finland: kids don't begin school until the age of seven, they rarely touch homework until they're teenagers, and there's only *one* mandatory standard-

ized test—taken when they're sixteen. How do the Finns do? They consistently score in the top 5 of global educational rankings (such as Pearson's *Learning Curve*), which is why we see books like *Finnish Lessons: What Can the World Learn from Educational Change in Finland?*

Children of America: you're welcome.*

Apologizing

I'm sorry you have to read this. I'm sorry if this book isn't entertaining enough. I'm sorry you might not like certain parts. I'm sorry that I keep apologizing right now . . . Enough. Too many "I'm sorrys" can seem like drivel, they weaken us, and they could mask a deeper problem.

"A litany of apologies is something you need to look into," says psychiatrist Robert London. " 'I'm sorry I'm late' is perfect when you're late, but 'I'm sorry' when you're late every day doesn't cut it."

Studies have shown that women apologize more than men. "Our research suggests that men and women have different thresholds for what constitutes offensive behavior—women have a lower threshold for behavior they find offensive or bothersome," psychologist Dr. Karina Schumann tells me. "This suggests that women

---

*Methodologies matter. Pope says that some of the studies simply look at the correlation of homework with GPA, which is a tad definitional, as grades are often pegged directly to homework. It's a tautology. This is why different studies yield different results, and homework enthusiasts have their own set of data to cheer.

apologize more frequently (at least in part) because they find more behaviors offensive. But when men do think they have committed an offense, they appear to be just as likely to apologize as women." Or, put less elegantly, we men don't realize when we're being pricks.

I know I'm an overapologizer. What should I do? I ask Dr. Schumann for suggestions on how I can change, and she suggests keeping a daily diary of my apologies. I love this idea: a Sorry Journal. "Every time you catch yourself apologizing, jot it down in your smartphone or notepad," she advises. "Write down what happened, why you thought an apology was necessary, and whether the apology helped."

The first morning, here are some of my many, many apologies:

"Sorry!" I say this in the office hallways again and again. Not just when I bump into someone, but when there's even the slightest possibility of contact. This makes no sense. I make a mental note to swap "I'm sorry" for "Excuse me."

"Sorry, I think you have the wrong number," I say to the person who called, even though *he* is the one who made the mistake.

I was supposed to go on a date that night and the woman canceled on me. Her text: "Don't hate me but I think I have to raincheck tonight. I'm not feeling very good . . ." My response: "Sorry you're not feeling well . . ." The Sorry Journal forced me to realize that *she* is the one who canceled and *I* am the one who apologized.

The implications of this text troubled me, so I did a search for the word "sorry" across all my texts. The results filled me with shame: I kept scrolling . . . and scrolling . . . and scrolling. Literally hundreds of texts. To friends, family, dates. They all began to look the same.

- "Hey, Happy Birthday! I'm sorry I couldn't make it—"
- "Sorry I missed your call!"
- "Sorry I won't be there—"
- "Sorry about your shoes, that's a bummer."
- "Sorry!"
- "Yeah, sorry I've been totally out of the loop on this—"

And on and on and on.

A few patterns emerged. One is that I constantly apologize for things that don't require an apology. This is dumb. The second is that I apologize so much, so effusively, that my apologies have lost their punch, and whenever I *really* need to apologize, either my usual apology is now just white noise or, sometimes, I feel the need to go over the top with an even grander apology.

For example, on the first morning of my Sorry Journal, when I responded to an e-mail from someone I hadn't met personally, I wrote, "Thanks again, sir." That's normally a harmless sentence. Except I got this reply minutes later: ":) quick note—it's Ms. Brett Ford." Oh shit. I just assumed the person was a male, which was both lazy and sexist, and while I don't mind being lazy, I hate being sexist. I was appalled. I wrote back, "I am MORTIFIED. Please accept my apologies, sorry, Brett." Apologies are like any drug, and when you do it too much, you need an even bigger dose to feel the same impact.

The third pattern, though, is even more unsettling. I was chronically apologizing for being late, for failing to return a text, for not calling someone back, for missing someone's birthday. This didn't happen just occasionally. It's *constant*. I had replaced *being there* with *sorry I'm not there*. I love all my family and friends. But

maybe I've spread myself too thin, let them down, or taken them for granted. This is yet another sneaky downside of apologies: they mask what's really going on. When I say "I'm sorry," I'm letting myself off the hook (in the same way that we let ourselves off the hook when we buy organic gummy bears). Instead of apologizing, the correct action is to think about what you've done, then think about it some more, and then take measures to ensure it won't happen again. Which, up until now, I have failed to do.

And for that, I am sorry.

Multitasking

I just did a quick search on Monster.com for jobs that require multitasking. It fetched over 1,000 postings— assistants, vice presidents, nurses, graphic designers—with requirements like "multitasking of multiple projects are essential for this role." We're multitasking junkies. We crave it. At work we're expected to do seven things at once. At home we scroll through Instagram while texting our friends while watching TV on our "second-screen experience." At Starbucks, we no longer simply wait in line while collecting our thoughts, and we would certainly never do the unthinkable—talk to strangers—instead we listen to our podcasts while checking our e-mail while live-tweeting a photo of the barista's purple beard.

But what's the cost of this whipsawing from task to task?

The gold standard of multitasking research is the work of Stanford professor Clifford Nass, who, before he passed away in 2013, conducted a series of tests for both heavy multitaskers and light multitaskers. The back-and-forth switchers performed worse in

every possible way. For example, they were flashed a mix of images that had both letters and numbers, and then told to ignore the letters, focus on the numbers, and press a button if the number is even, and a different button if the number is odd. The multitaskers kept getting distracted by the letters and pressing the wrong buttons. Sloppy mistakes like this happened in test after test. "It turns out multitaskers are terrible at every aspect of multitasking," Nass said in a 2010 interview. "They're terrible at ignoring irrelevant information; they're terrible at keeping information in their head nicely and neatly organized; and they're terrible at switching from one task to another."

But it gets worse. Toggling back and forth between e-mail and Excel and PowerPoint doesn't just sap your productivity in the moment; it may take a long-term toll on your brain. "Our brains have to be retrained to multitask. . . . We train our brains to a new way of thinking," said Nass. But when we try to go back, we find that "our brains are plastic but they're not elastic. They don't just snap back into shape." Can this be undone? The jury is out. Nass attempted to conduct an experiment that studied the brains of heavy multitaskers who went cold turkey for two weeks, but he couldn't round up enough volunteers—they just couldn't quit.

Multitasking causes stress. Dr. Gloria Mark, a professor of informatics at UC Irvine, hooked up college students with heart-rate monitors, then studied the impact of social media and multitasking. "With more window-switches, the higher the stress," she writes in the study. It's obvious that multitasking can be distracting. Less obvious is that it can strain our "cognitive load" and put too much pressure on our brain to juggle the competing tasks. "Switching windows frequently to a completely different site

(e.g., from Facebook to an academic site) could also increase cognitive load, as one needs to continually reorient," Mark writes.

I'm a weak man. I easily bend to the addiction of Alt-Tab, so the only way I get things done is to physically remove the temptation. I use a program called Freedom to sever my laptop from the Internet, then I take my iPhone and banish it from the room, even stowing it in a locker. (In psychiatry this is known as a "Ulysses pact": knowing that he would be lured to his death by the song of the Sirens, Ulysses ordered his men to strap him to the mast to avoid temptation.) I felt a little less stupid when I learned that other writers do the same thing; when George R. R. Martin sits down to kill off the Starks, he does so on an offline 1990s-era DOS computer. And as Jonathan Franzen once said in a bit of hyperbole, "It's doubtful that anyone with an Internet connection at his workplace is writing good fiction." Franzen went even further, gutting his computer of its Internet card and sealing the ethernet port.

Inevitably, though, I'll get back online and tell myself that I need to "multitask" to do research and answer e-mails. Like today. It took me three times as long to write this topic as it should, as I checked Facebook five times, posted a few tweets, checked e-mail seven times, and read a long-form piece about the career of Steven Soderbergh. Because of course.

Eye contact

We all know the stereotype: the guy who doesn't make eye contact is a wimp. Or he has something to hide. We associate strong

eye contact with a manly man's self-confidence, persuasion, and the dreamy gaze of Ryan Gosling.

But too much eye contact, just like too much homework, can backfire.

In a 2013 study in Germany, scientists used something called "eye-tracking technology" to monitor the pupils of a group of volunteers. These volunteers then watched a range of persuasive speeches—some of the speakers made strong eye contact, some did not. They found the opposite of what you might expect: when the presenters held eye contact, the viewers were less likely to change their minds. "There is a lot of cultural lore about the power of eye contact as an influence tool," said researcher Frances Chen. "But our findings show that direct eye contact makes skeptical listeners less likely to change their minds, not more, as previously believed."

I reached out to the undisputed queen of eye contact and body language, Dr. Carol Goman, who jets around the world to give lectures at companies like GE and 3M. Her research has found that eye contact—and preferences about eye contact—varies between men and women. "Men simply don't need that kind of sustained eye contact; in fact, they don't need it at a very young age," she says. "Mothers tell me that the only time they talk to their teenage sons is when they're driving, and they can't have eye contact." So if a girlfriend, say, is trying to engage her boyfriend in a Big Serious Talk, Goman says it's more effective to sit side-by-side. "He might be more comfortable explaining his feelings if you don't demand eye contact."

Eye contact still has its place. It's still true that in the getting-to-know-you phase, stronger eye contact helps win friends and

influence people. Goman even has a handy trick for gauging exactly how long you should hold someone's gaze in the workplace: "A simple way to enhance positive eye contact is to look in their eyes long enough to make a mental note of the eye color of everyone you meet. You don't have to remember the color, just gaze long enough to notice it. With this one exercise, you will dramatically increase your likeability factor."

Happiness

The ultimate paradox: trying to be happy might make you less happy. "Feeling happy feels good, and tends to be good for you, too. However, *wanting* to feel happy may work against us," says researcher Brett Ford.* Her studies suggest that when people actively try hard to be happy, this somehow works against them. "For example, we've found that people who are extremely motivated to feel happiness (who endorse ideas like, 'if I don't feel happy, maybe there's something wrong with me' or 'to have a meaningful life, I need to feel happy most of the time') are more likely to experience severe mood disorder symptoms, like depression and mania." The concept is almost Zen: the more we chase the Lady of Happiness, the more likely she is to elude us. Maybe it's better to just *Be*.

Some of this might have to do with lofty expectations. When we get hell-bent on pursuing happiness, we create an impossible goal that reality can never match. Ford also suspects that "when

---

*If that name sounds familiar, yes, she was polite enough to react good-naturedly to my "Thank you, sir!" e-mail.

people monitor their own happiness all the time, the very act of constantly paying attention to their own happiness can hinder the ability to feel happy."

Yale researcher June Gruber considers all this in her study "A Dark Side of Happiness? How, When, and Why Happiness Is Not Always Good." Her team asks four questions:

1. Is there a wrong degree of happiness?
2. Is there a wrong time for happiness?
3. Are there wrong ways to pursue happiness?
4. Are there wrong types of happiness?

The short answers are yes, yes, yes, and yes. For the first question, *degree of happiness,* this once again goes back to dosage and the Greek Golden Mean, which holds that too much of anything is unhealthy—even happiness. "Meta-analytic data suggest that at a very high intensity of happiness, people experience no psychological or health gains and sometimes they experience costs," writes Gruber. Other research has found that when we're exuberantly happy, we're more likely to throw caution to the wind and make poor decisions. (Example: Never ask your financial planner for advice on the day she wins the lottery.) "One manic may give away his life's savings on a whim, while another joyfully drives 100 mph to a sexual liaison with a potentially dangerous stranger," notes researcher Dr. Randolph M. Nesse from Arizona State University.

Other studies have found an inverse relationship between happiness and creativity. (It's not a coincidence that so many artists are tortured souls.) And as we see in *Happy,* 2011's little-indie-that-could documentary, too many of us pursue money, careers, and

BMWs instead of the simpler, more altruistic values that nourish the soul.

Even by the standards of this book, pinning down happiness is an absurdly large task; essentially, it's the thread that runs through the last three thousand years of philosophy. As Aristotle said, "Happiness is the meaning and the purpose of life, the whole aim and end of human existence." I don't think we'll solve the issue in these two pages. This shortcoming makes me a little unhappy, but I suppose that's for the best.

Meditation

In a meta-study of forty-seven trials and over 3,000 participants, the American Medical Association found that meditation had only "low evidence" of improved quality of life and "low evidence or no effect" on positive mood, eating habits, sleep, and weight.

And then there's this. In some of the most intense bouts of meditation, it's possible that the brain itself is subtly transformed, and that this transformation can sabotage our ability to understand the physical reality around us. This has to do with *losing our sense of self.*

"In a meditation practice where a person says, 'I've lost my sense of self,' when that's the goal, that can be an *amazing* experience," Dr. Andrew Newberg, the director of research at the Myrna Brind Center of Integrative Medicine, tells me. "But if it's somebody with moderate or severe psychological issues, where the sense of self is a little tenuous to begin with, then losing your sense of self can be traumatic."

He's actually found a way to measure this, scanning the brains of

meditators. With intense meditation, Newberg found a decline in blood flowing to the brain's posterior superior parietal lobe, which governs our spatial relationship. "We know that the posterior superior parietal lobe plays that particular role because there are patients with damage in this same region who literally cannot move around without falling," Newberg told *The Humanist*. "They'll miss the chair they intended to sit on, and generally have a fuzzy understanding of where their body ends and the rest of the universe begins."

In fairness, this is not a reason to avoid meditation. "These are pretty rare," he assures me. "Millions of people have meditated, and there's a limited number of these types of reports—a handful." Or as our framework would say, *the absolute risk is low*. And meditation almost certainly lowers the absolute risk of many other things, such as health problems related to stress.

A more legitimate downside? It's not for everyone. "If somebody tries the practice and doesn't really like it, and it just doesn't make sense to them, then they feel funny doing it," says Newberg. "This can be frustrating to people. It can be upsetting if you're doing the wrong practice for you."

I have no quarrel with meditation. Millions of people swear by it. Many, many, many other studies have linked it with countless health benefits, and I like the principle of cutting away life's noise and focusing on what matters. Saying meditation is bad is like saying *thinking* is bad.

Self-Help Books

Each year, roughly five thousand self-help books are published. They dominate the bestseller lists. Thousands of self-help websites,

blogs, online forums, and apps are a click away. But do they work?

"There is no relationship between the quality of the self-help book and its status as a bestseller," says Dr. John Norcross, a professor of psychology at the University of Scranton, who, for twenty years, has led a team of researchers analyzing the merits of self-help resources. "We've done tests. The correlation is zero."

I didn't think this sort of thing was testable, but they've conducted experiments to gauge the books' efficacy: You round up a bunch of depressed people, and you randomly assign one group to read a self-help book, and then a control group to read a novel. Then you do a follow-up to see if they feel better. According to Norcross, there are only about a dozen self-help books that have undergone such trials. Over 99.9 percent of self-help books are never tested before going to market. This can cause problems. He ticks off the potential downsides:

1. Inaccurate diagnosis. It's easy to read a book's introduction and think it applies to you—a general list of symptoms can apply to anyone, like a horoscope—but if you've misdiagnosed the problem, the rest of the book is useless.

2. Inaccurate information and ineffective methods. "Anyone can write a self-help book," he says, pointing out that the author of *The Secret*, Rhonda Byrne, was a television producer. "*The Secret* says that you can physically manipulate reality with your mind. That everyone is responsible for everything that happens to them—including cancer patients, rape victims." After calling bullshit on

The Secret on morning shows, he received both hate mail
and letters of thanks.

3. A sense of hopelessness. If the self-help books don't work,
people think they've already given treatment a shot—but
they haven't, really—and are then less likely to seek
proper help.

4. Death. The charismatic guru James Arthur Ray, author
of *Harmonic Wealth: The Secret of Attracting the Life You
Want,* held a "Spiritual Warrior" retreat in an Arizona
sweat lodge. He asked people to fast. Three of them died.

It's no surprise to hear that *The Secret* was panned by the experts, but they also gave low marks to *Men Are from Mars, Women
Are from Venus.* "The majority of psychologists do not think well
of that book, which oversimplifies relationships," Norcross says.
Over the past twenty years, he created something of a Rotten-
Tomatoes.com for self-help books, sending surveys to a network of
roughly five thousand psychologists, asking them to rank a given
self-help book (or website, blog, etc.) on the following scale:

Extremely good: +2
Moderately good: +1
Average: 0
Moderately bad: -1
Extremely bad: -2

These survey responses feed a monster dataset, which allows his
team to aggregate the scores and make generalizations about how,
on average, the resources stacked up. He shares the results in his

book *Self-Help That Works*. For self-help books, with a sample size of 760, these were the findings:

Very helpful: 27 percent
Somewhat helpful: 58 percent
No effect: 8 percent
Somewhat harmful: 5 percent
Very harmful: 2 percent

At first blush, this looks pretty solid: 85 percent are either somewhat or very helpful. Not too shabby. Then again, would you eat a food if you knew there was a 7 percent chance it was somewhat or very harmful? Would you a drink a gallon of milk that's slapped with the label warning: 7 percent chance the milk is rotten? Milk is regulated. Drugs are regulated. Norcross raises a provocative point: yes, self-help books are protected by the First Amendment, but in essence *they are medicine*. Unregulated medicine. Self-medicate with discretion.

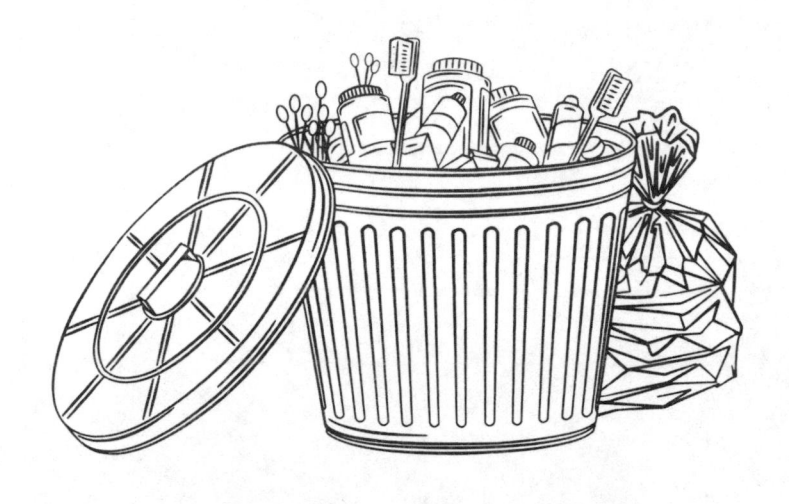

MEDICINE

Some people are obsessed with staying current on the latest trends in medical care, seeing a doctor at the first sign of trouble and never skipping their annual physical. Then there's the rest of us. So if you're something of a medicine slacker, this should cheer you up.

Multivitamins

In 1954, a scientist named Linus Pauling won the Nobel Prize in Chemistry. Something of an overachiever, he followed this up by winning a *second* Nobel Prize—this time for Peace. The man could do no wrong. In the 1970s he turned his eyes toward a juicy new field: vitamins. He published the book *Vitamin C and the Common Cold,* convinced that gobs of vitamin C could save us from colds, heart disease, arthritis, asthma, cancer, and everything from kidney failure to AIDS.

People listened. And why shouldn't they? Dr. Pauling was a living legend, a god. He said we should take a dose of 3,000 milligrams a day—about thirty times the recommended daily allowance—and he personally swallowed 18,000 milligrams a day.

According to many doctors, there was only one problem with Pauling's theories: they were all wrong. Pauling was afflicted with "Nobel disease," a condition where a master in one field thinks he's an authority in others, according to Dr. Steven Salzberg, professor of medicine and biostatistics at Johns Hopkins, and a frequent debunker of pseudoscience. "He wasn't an expert in nutrition. He was just completely wrong about this. All the evidence says he's wrong."

But by then it didn't really matter, as he had sowed the seeds for the $32 billion multivitamin industry. Half of all adults in the United States pop a daily multivitamin. "All of us have this notion

that if something is necessary to your health, then you should have a lot of it, right? But that's just not true!" Salzberg says, laughing. "Our body needs a balance. And vitamins? We only need a tiny bit."

We do need vitamins. Just ask Columbus: if we don't have vitamin C we get scurvy. But nowadays we get plenty through our food. Taking twenty times the required vitamin C is about as useful as, say, carrying twenty umbrellas to stay dry.

In 2013, a team of doctors sifted through the results of twenty-seven different trials that assessed the efficacy of multivitamins—with a combined sample size of four hundred thousand adults—and tracked six thousand men over the course of twelve years. Their findings? In the scientist equivalent of a WWF wrestler throwing a chair across the ring, they called their study "Enough Is Enough: Stop Wasting Money on Vitamin and Mineral Supplements." They found zero long-term benefits if you take multivitamins. None.

"The [vitamin and supplement] industry is based on anecdote, people saying, 'I take this, and it makes me feel better,'" wrote a coauthor of the study, Dr. Edgar Miller. "It's perpetuated. But when you put it to the test, there's no evidence of benefit in the long term. It can't prevent mortality, stroke or heart attack."

Not every doctor agrees. The Harvard School of Public Health, for example, suggests that a daily pill can be a useful hedge. "For those who eat a healthy diet, a multivitamin may have little or no benefit. . . . But not everyone manages to eat a healthful diet. . . . For these reasons, we believe a daily multivitamin-multimineral pill offers safe, simple micronutrient insurance." Another key rebuttal: it's also possible that multivitamins have a positive effect that's more subtle than "lowering the mortality rates." Maybe they

help boost your energy, give you an extra kick at the gym, or improve the complexion of your skin. None of these nuanced effects would be captured in a long-term study of mortality rates or heart attacks. Or maybe, for some people, multivitamins are like an atheist who prays to God, just in case—what's the harm, right?

I pressed Salzberg on this issue. What if you never, ever eat any broccoli or carrots, living on the Taco Bell diet? (This was basically my junk cleanse.) Maybe then you'd be better off with a multivitamin?

"That's not a healthy way to live," he says.

"Right, but *if* someone refuses to eat a balanced diet, could multivitamins help fill the gaps?"

"I wouldn't give that as general advice to people. A lot of people eat a very unhealthy diet, but they're fooling themselves to think they can eat burgers and fries and not fruits and vegetables, and then take a multivitamin. The vitamin industry relies upon that."

"Right, but if someone—for whatever dumb reason—refuses to eat healthy, is there maybe a benefit?" (In fairness to Dr. Salzberg, who wasn't part of the study, now I'm being a bit of a jerk.)

He pauses. "If someone *refuses* to eat healthy, then . . . maybe."

Pop your pills accordingly.

Annual Physicals

My dad gives good advice. In my twenties, as I swung from vine to vine in the jungle that is freelance writing, he encouraged me

to sock away money in an IRA (even when it felt impossible), keep some form of health insurance (even before it was mandatory), and "Be sure to get your annual physical."

This seems sensible. Prudent. It fits neatly in our American ethos of personal accountability, preventative maintenance, and an ideology of better safe than sorry.

But new research says that it might be a waste of time.

In 2013, Danish scientists analyzed the results of sixteen studies across roughly 185,000 people, hunting for evidence that regular checkups translated into rosier health, well-being, or longevity. They found none. The researchers compared two groups: patients with regular checkups and patients who saw their doctors only when they felt like it. The routine visits seemed to make no difference. "The study adds to growing evidence that periodic exams in otherwise healthy adults are a waste of money and may even lead to overdiagnosis and unnecessary treatments," said the lead researcher, Dr. Lasse Krogsboll of the Nordic Cochrane Centre in Copenhagen.*

That study had precedent. In 1979, after reaching similar conclusions from similar studies, the Canadian government recommended that doctors abandon the practice of annual physicals. "Faced with such evidence, I have not gotten an annual physical since around the time I finished my medical training in 1989," writes Elisabeth Rosenthal in a piece called 'Let's (Not) Get

---

* This meta-study was of the epidemiological ilk, meaning that we can't really parse correlation and causation. By now, I'm pretty sure there's a correlation between the number of times I say "correlation versus causation" and the number of times you roll your eyes, although we can't tell for sure if that link is causal.

Physicals.' for *The New York Times*. "I respect my doctors, but I see them only when I'm sick. I religiously follow schedules for the limited number of screening tests recommended for women my age—like mammograms every two years and blood pressure checks—but most of those do not require a special office visit."

Rosenthal cites a doctor who doesn't believe in automatic annual checkups for every patient, Dr. Allan Brett, who has both A) thirty-five years of primary care internal medicine experience, and B) an academic interest in doctor-patient relationships. I tracked him down for additional insight. "To take the most extreme view, and say that every person must have a head-to-toe evaluation every year—it's nonsense," Brett tells me. He cautioned that no clinical studies have emphatically proven the case one way or the other, but suspects that "If you *did* subject that to a randomized trial, it's hard for me to believe that the outcome would be better in the annual physical group."

Brett explains that most physicians are either in the Less Is More camp or the More Is More, and he tends to skew to the former. "When we do lots of testing in people without symptoms, we do find some results that are slightly outside of the usual range, but the vast majority of these abnormalities are meaningless—we call them false positives. There are downstream harms of testing everybody and finding lots of false positives."

These "downstream harms" include anxiety that is often unwarranted. And then more tests, then more tests, then more tests—which do little more than reassure the patient. "The test might say that you're a couple of a tenths of a point above the normal range. There's no need to treat it when it's barely above the normal range, and some people will just obsess over that," Brett says. "Or if you do a panel of twenty or forty tests, it's actually quite

likely that at least *one* of the results will be outside the range of normal." Statistically speaking, it's abnormal to have zero abnormalities, but this is tough for doctors to convey in a twenty-minute session.

Brett is quick to point out that this isn't a universal guideline, and his philosophy varies by patient. Context matters. The strategy for a healthy twenty-five-year-old woman is different from a seventy-three-year-old with chronic medical problems.

From a policy perspective, the issue is far more complicated. Trade-offs abound. There's no consensus. One group argues that by encouraging all citizens to have annual physicals, we'll catch problems that would later cost the taxpayers billions; others argue that while physicals matter for some people, millions of them are a waste of resources.

Takeaway: Hey, Doc, see ya in 2027! (Kidding. Sort of.)

Aspirin

Aspirin is good for your heart. Aspirin causes ulcers. It's good. It's bad. It reminds me of an old joke that my high school economics teacher liked to tell: "Why is it a good idea to cut off an economist's hand? Because they're always saying, 'On the one hand, on the other hand . . .'"

The problem is that all of these things are true. The conventional wisdom is that aspirin is good for your heart, which is why, in the United States alone, 40 million of us pop a daily aspirin. Plenty of studies suggest that aspirin trims the risk of colon cancer, pancreatic cancer, and heart attacks. But other studies have pegged aspirin to

higher risks of internal bleeding and hemorrhagic strokes. Which means that we should do . . . what, exactly?

The trade-off is nicely framed on Harvard Medical School's site: "Aspirin suppresses the formation of blood clots, the villains behind heart attacks and most strokes. But in doing so, aspirin boosts the risk for bleeding in the stomach and brain. The critical question is whether the risk of cardiovascular disease outweighs the risk of bleeding. Right now, the answer is not simple."

Even one of the plum studies that shows the merits of aspirin, published in *The Lancet*, uses language that's maddeningly back-and-forth. The abstract begins: "Daily aspirin reduces the long-term risk of death due to cancer." Okay, now we're talking! Firm. Decisive. Conclusive. The very next sentence: "However, the short-term effect is less certain, especially in women, effects on cancer incidence are largely unknown, and the time course of risk and benefit in primary prevention is unclear." Riiiiiight.

A 2013 analysis from Britain's University of Warwick found that when people used aspirin, the risk of internal bleeding spiked by 37 percent and the risk of hemorrhagic stroke increased by 38 percent. "Too many healthy people think that aspirin will prevent heart attacks and cancer," Dr. Peter Sandercock, commenting on the study, said to the *Telegraph*. "This shows that if you are healthy, with no symptoms of cardiovascular disease, then it is not sensible to take regular aspirin. It won't improve your health." And like a two-handed economist, he adds that on the other hand, if you *do* have a higher risk of heart attack or stroke—especially if you've already had one—this changes the math, tilting the odds in favor of aspirin. "Aspirin could reduce the stroke risk by one quarter, and that big benefit outweighs the small bleeding risk."

Another complicating factor about trade-offs: "The benefits and harms of trade-offs are often very modest on either side," says Dr. David Tovey, the editor in chief of the Cochrane Library, based in Britain, whose voice is a dead ringer for Sir Alec Guinness. "I was listening to a radio program the other day, and a member of Parliament talked about how whether people have access to a new drug is *the difference between life and death.*" The drug in question was Herceptin, which treats breast cancer. "It's a good drug. It's an effective drug. But that doesn't mean that everyone who takes it will survive breast cancer." He explains that out of one hundred people who take the drug, eight might not have a recurrence *anyway*, but that sixteen wouldn't have a recurrence if they take the drug. So the only people affected by the drug are those incremental eight—or 8 percent of the population. "That's much less than the idea that if you take it you'll live, you don't take it you'll die, which is often the basis of reporting."

This is giving me a headache. I'm taking an aspirin.

Mammograms

Roughly one in eight women will develop breast cancer. In the United States alone, there are an estimated 2.8 million women who are either currently being treated or have been treated. I have a friend with breast cancer. Most of us do. It's scary. It's awful. So it was something of a shock when, in 2009, a task force from the U.S. Department of Health changed the guidelines of mammogram screenings—from once every year to once every two years. The specific recommendations, as WebMD lays it out:

- Routine screening of average-risk women should begin at age fifty, instead of age forty.
- Routine screening should end at age seventy-four.
- Women should get screening mammograms every two years instead of every year.
- Breast self-exams have little value, based on findings from several large studies.

"Annual screening is associated with a greater likelihood of false positive results, which have an adverse impact on women's well-being and quality of life," said the study's lead researcher, Dr. Laura J. Esserman of UC San Francisco. The logic: if there's no incremental value in screening annually as opposed to biannually, this could save roughly $7.8 billion in costs, which could be allocated to other areas of women's health. "We could increase women's participation in screening, improve routine assessment of breast cancer risk and referral services for women at high risk, offer better genetic counseling for women with a family history of breast cancer and work on improving the quality of screening, with an emphasis on higher-quality mammography read by specialized mammographers."

But why, exactly, has the annual screening fallen out of favor? Are they suddenly more dangerous? Or was annual screening never as effective as we thought? "Simply finding cancer is not proof of a test's benefit. One must find the cancer, provide treatment, and demonstrate that patients who would have died do not. Several screening tests for other cancers have been found not just useless but also harmful because the nature of the cancer was that early detection and treatment did not save lives," explains CNN's

Dr. Otis Brawley, chief medical officer of the American Cancer Society.

A more recent study (2014) points to a similar conclusion, but one that's even more provocative, suggesting that *any* mammograms, regardless of frequency, had little or no ability to save lives. This is unsettling and difficult to explain. Over a period of twenty-five years, Canadian researchers tracked forty-five thousand women between the ages of forty and fifty-nine, and then compared them to a control group of forty-five thousand women who were instructed not to get screening. In both panels, about five hundred women died from breast cancer. The screenings seemed to have no impact. "And the screening had harms: One in five cancers found with mammography and treated was not a threat to the woman's health and did not need treatment such as chemotherapy, surgery or radiation," writes Gina Kolata. The takeaway isn't that "ignorance is bliss." It's the opposite. The researchers theorize that it's *precisely because* women are better educated—and take drugs like tamoxifen, which have lowered the death rates—that mammograms are less relevant than in the old days.

This is an excellent place to remind you that I am as close to being a doctor as Vin Diesel is to being a nuclear engineer, so please, talk to a trained professional.

Teeth Brushing

C'mon, *really*? Is nothing sacred? You're telling me that brushing our goddamn teeth can be bad for us?

Sometimes. As writer Jennifer Berman discovered in her infamous epiphany "Kale? Juicing? Trouble Ahead," the natural acids

in her fruit and vegetable juices—carrots, celery, lemons—had eroded the enamel in her teeth, and she only made the problem worse by brushing immediately after. Apparently this is a no-no.

Baffled, I asked my own dentist to help set me straight. Dr. Nancy Rojas, a lovely woman who has helped me with root canals, warns that if you brush too soon after a meal, "the acid will soften the enamel, and this will cause you to 'brush off' enamel." This doesn't mean that you need to skip a brush. If you want to brush immediately after, Rojas suggests first rinsing your mouth with water, as this will dilute the acids and lessen the chance that they'll be mashed into your teeth.

Bonus tip? "Eating cheese will neutralize the acid and save the erosion of your enamel." (Hey, cheese industry: here's a billion-dollar idea for you: a marketing campaign that trumpets the benefit of cheese to our teeth, which gives us a nice white smile. Tagline? "Say 'Cheese.'")

This doesn't give us license to skip. And the last thing we should do is skip our nighttime brushing, which Rojas sees many patients do, as they (mistakenly) assume that the morning brushing is the one that really counts. They've got it backwards. "It's most important to brush before bed. Your accumulation from an entire day of eating will sit in your teeth overnight. Bacteria breed and will have a party in your mouth." Saliva is your friend. During the day, it works to keep your teeth and gums moist, and this constant flow will keep your teeth clean(ish). At night? "Your salivary flow decreases, so the bad bacteria have an opportunity to sit still and cause damage."

Following in the book's spirit of how too much of anything can be unhealthy, *brushing too hard* can cause problems. "Brushing hard also causes extreme damage because it wears out your enamel,"

says Rojas. "Enamel is the hardest substance in your body, but the daily hard 'scrubbing' motion can cause enamel abrasion. Therefore a soft bristle brush is always recommended. Nonabrasive toothpaste." And in a blow to the All-Natural-All-The-Timers, she cautions, "Some natural ones may be too harsh."

So consult your dentist before buying Organic Thoreau Toothpaste.

Statins

File this under Bad News About What's Good for You, but Screw it, You Probably Need to Keep Doing it Anyway.

People who take statins (drugs that lower cholesterol) do it to prevent heart attacks. These are also probably people who need to exercise. So for the millions of people on statins, it was something of a bummer when a 2013 study found that, well, statins might completely negate whatever benefits you get from exercise.

This seems to be a good study. It's a clinical one, not epidemiological. Researchers from the University of Missouri split a group of overweight men and women with high blood pressure into two groups, and had both groups exercise for twelve weeks. One group took Zocor. One group did not. The group that did *not* take the statin improved their fitness levels by 10 percent (measured by ability to jog on a treadmill). The statin-poppers? After these twelve weeks of exercise, they *only improved their fitness by 1 percent*. One. Frickin'. Percent. (Coincidentally, that's the same rate of improvement from a low-sodium diet.)

"Why there should be such a discrepancy between the two groups' fitness levels wasn't clear on the surface," writes Gretchen

Reynolds. "But when the researchers looked microscopically at bi-opsied muscle tissue, they found notable differences in the levels of an enzyme related to the health of mitochondria, the tiny energy-producing parts of a cell. Mitochondria generally increase in number and potency when someone exercises." In the control group, during the three months of exercise, the jogging led to a 13 percent boost in mitochondria-enzyme levels. This is good. But for the statin-poppers, the mitochondria-enzymes actually fell by 4.5 percent. This is bad. And it might help explain one well-documented side effect of statins: that they can cause muscle aches and pains.

So, the takeaway? Frustrating as hell. Despite the results, the experts still recommended that at-risk people (high cholesterol, history of heart problems) continue to take statins and that they continue to exercise. Just try to ignore the fact that, well, maybe it's not doing a damn bit of good.

On to something lighter . . .

Q-tips

"Breathe in. Now breathe out," my doctor tells me.

I do so. I'm naked except for my underwear and a hospital gown. Annual physical time! (This is before I learned that maybe I don't need annual physicals.) I tell my doctor about the premise of the book, and I ask him for his favorite example of something we commonly think of as "good for us" that actually has a dark side.

"Q-tips," he says, checking my posture.

"Pushing them in your ears too hard?"

"Using them at all. You don't need them."

But . . . but . . . "Don't we need to clean our ears?"

"All Q-tips do is push the wax inside your ear. They're worthless."

Huh. I later did a little research and found that, sure enough, once again, what I was taught in third grade was dead wrong. The key takeaway: ear wax is good for you. We can just let it be. We *should* just let it be. According to the official guidelines for the American Academy of Otolaryngology (only seventeen people have ever spoken the word "otolaryngology"), "Cerumen, commonly called 'earwax,' is not really a 'wax' but a water-soluble mixture of secretions (produced in the outer third of the ear canal), plus hair and dead skin, that serves a protective function for the ear. Cerumen is a natural product that should not be routinely removed unless impacted. . . . Cerumen is a beneficial, self-cleaning agent, with protective, lubricating (emollient), and antibacterial properties." Every year, about 8 million people go to their doctors for a cerumen-removal procedure, and a good chunk of those—no one knows the number—were caused by people using Q-tips.

As *Slate*'s William Brennan observes, even the official website for Q-tips recommends that you should "stroke . . . gently around the outer ear, *without entering the ear canal*." (Italics are mine.) He also found that the word "ear" appears only eight times on the entire Q-tip website, which tends to encourage other applications like "cleaning the small crevices of your dog or cat's face."

The best way to clean your ears? Eat food. It really is that simple. When we move our jaws, the motion shakes the old earwax free—it's so subtle we can't feel it or see it—and it tumbles to the ground. Done and done. This happens whether we're eating or

talking. So if you're someone who never eats food and never says a word, then it's possible you might need Q-tips. Everyone else doesn't.

Exhibit A: Hannah, from *Girls*. If you watch the show, you might remember a scene where Lena Dunham, crippled by OCD, plunges a Q-tip deep into her ear and then races to the hospital. It's painful to watch. As Dunham later tweeted, "If all I've done on this earth is scare you out of using Q-tips, I will die a happy and purposeful woman."

Blood Pressure Drugs

Roughly one out of every three Americans has high blood pressure. It's a more serious problem when we get older, like nostril hair. It can be deadly. If you flip open a medical textbook and point at a random disease, chances are it can be caused by high blood pressure—it ups the risk of aneurisms, strokes, dementia, kidney failure, heart attacks, bone loss, sleep apnea, death.

So medication usually makes sense. And according to the CDC, about 76 percent of adults with high blood pressure are taking medication like Lopressor and Tenoretic. But a gloomy study in 2014 showed that when the elderly take this type of medication, they are more likely to fall. That's not trivial. Falls lead to hip fractures, and for the elderly, when you break your hip, your short-term mortality rate doubles. (Alas, there is no "good news" about hip fractures.)

Here's how the study worked:

About five thousand elderly (average age of eighty) were tracked for three years.

People who took no medication: 7.5 percent had a serious injury from a fall.

People who took moderate intensity medication: 9.8 percent.

People who took high-intensity medication: 8.2 percent

So it's by no means a guarantee that someone will fall (the *absolute risk* is still relatively low), but in the world of health studies, the difference between 7.5 and 8.2—the relative risk—is statistically significant. It's an observational study, so there's no way to untwine correlation from causation. But this does square with what many doctors suspect; as the study's coauthor, Dr. Mary E. Tinetti, told *Reuters*, "Clinically, it is not uncommon for an older adult to say that they think their blood pressure medications are making them feel dizzy or weak or unsteady."

What does this mean? Should we be taking this damn medication or not? As is often the case, there's no clear-cut answer. It's a matter of juggling the risks. "It is probably the case that some older adults are at greater risk of having a stroke and controlling their blood pressure is in their best interest," said Tinetti, suggesting that for them, the absolute risk from high blood pressure outweighs the increase in relative risk of falls. "However, for others, the risk of a serious fall injury such as head injury or hip fracture may outweigh the benefit of blood pressure medications."

That kind of hemming-and-hawing makes you wonder, *Damn, is it even worth it? Should I even bother with new medical procedures?*

Glad you asked . . .

New Medical Procedures

Everyone has that crusty uncle who says, "I hate hospitals. Don't trust 'em. I'll heal just fine on my own."

Your uncle will be delighted by a 2013 study published in the *Mayo Clinic Proceedings*. The topic? Improvements in medical treatment. A team of scientists combed through ten years of studies from *The New England Journal of Medicine*—analyzing 363 studies in total—to answer a very simple question: What's better, the original treatment, or the new and "improved" treatment?

Here's what they found. New treatments were:

- No better or worse than the original: 40 percent
- Better than the original: 38 percent
- Inconclusive: 22 percent

What the hell? Isn't the field of medicine supposed to get better over time, like smartphones and Matthew McConaughey?

"Among the practices found to be ineffective or harmful were the routine use of hormone therapy in postmenopausal women; high-dose chemotherapy and stem cell transplant, a complex and expensive treatment for breast cancer that was found to be no better than conventional chemotherapy; and intensive glucose lowering in Type 2 diabetes patients in intensive care, which not only failed to reduce cardiovascular events but actually increased mortality," writes Nicholas Bakalar in *The New York Times*.

In fairness, of course, this tested new treatments versus original treatments, not new treatments versus no treatments. So your uncle can't claim a total triumph. One challenge is that in the

grand scheme of things—viewed through the prism of centuries and millennia, not months—our health care is pretty damn good. We've made big strides. Much of the important, low-hanging fruit of medicine (antibiotics, vaccines, calf implants) has already been plucked. Incremental gains are tough.

So for continued reading, I recommend your uncle pick up *How We Do Harm: A Doctor Breaks Ranks About Being Sick in America*, where Dr. Otis Brawley, the chief medical officer for the American Cancer Society, argues that our health care system is dysfunctional at best, doing harm at worst. Who's at fault? "I blame patients, I blame doctors, I blame hospitals, I blame drug companies, I blame insurance companies. Our health care system is messed up because the system is designed to fail, and everybody is responsible for health care failing as it is now."

It's the kind of sobering statement that just makes you want a drink. At least that's good for you.

Deodorant

Kidding—there's nothing bad about this. Please continue using it.

Herbal Supplements

At my local deli, just next to the gum and the Tic Tacs and the lip balm, you can find a smorgasbord of herbal supplements ("Horny Goat Weed!" "Weekend Prince!") that promise to boost your energy, make you happy, and restore your sexual vigor.

They boast that they're "all-natural!" Many of these supple-

ments have been "used for thousands of years" in other cultures. If it comes from the earth it must be safe, right? There's only one catch. Repeated studies have shown that most herbal supplements, to use precise scientific language, are a crock of shit. And they've cleverly eluded regulation from the FDA.

Dr. Donald Marcus, a professor at Baylor College of Medicine, has written extensively on the health dangers of herbal supplements. "The paradox is that many people are distrustful of the pharmaceutical industry, and they're concerned about what they put into their bodies," he tells me. "But instead of taking a well-defined compound that has been tested, they'll take a St. John's wort extract that contains probably *hundreds* of chemicals, and they have no idea what they're exposing themselves to."

Let's say you're a pharmaceutical company like Pfizer. When you bring a drug to market, you have the burden of proof to show the FDA that your medicine is rigorously tested, safe, and that it does what it says it does. But if you're selling an "herbal supplement," the burden of proof, for the most part, falls on the government to show that the pill is doing harm. So it's easier to make wild-ass claims.

Why the double standard?

Enter Orrin Hatch, who, as of this writing, is still the senior senator from Utah. In 1994, he pushed through the Dietary Supplement Health and Education Act, which, according to Marcus, is "arguably the worst bill in the history of health care regulation." Hatch's critics blame him for helping to create the "Silicon Valley of dietary supplements" in Utah, with these companies as key contributors to his election campaigns. "That law waved a wand over herbal extracts, which are used all over the world as medicines, to say that they are *not* medicines, and it exempts them from the usual FDA requirements."

As the Mayo Clinic lays it out: "Manufacturers don't have to seek FDA approval before putting dietary supplements on the market. In addition, companies can claim that products address a nutrient deficiency, support health or are linked to body functions—if they have supporting research and they include a disclaimer that the FDA hasn't evaluated the claim."

And this "supporting research" is often sketchy. No doubt some supplements are better than others, and it's certainly plausible that some are effective, but Marcus says that virtually no mainstream evidence exists to support their efficacy. "There's no evidence from reputable, independent sources that any of these herbal supplements have any benefit." The National Institutes of Health did studies of the most popular herbal supplements. None were found to be any better than a placebo.

"Basically, you can go to your garage and put together an ointment or tonic and sell it, and you can say it promotes heart health or sexual vigor," Marcus says. "They're wolves in sheep's clothing."

And it's one more reminder that "natural" doesn't always mean "healthy." Dog shit is all-natural. This doesn't mean it will give you an erection.

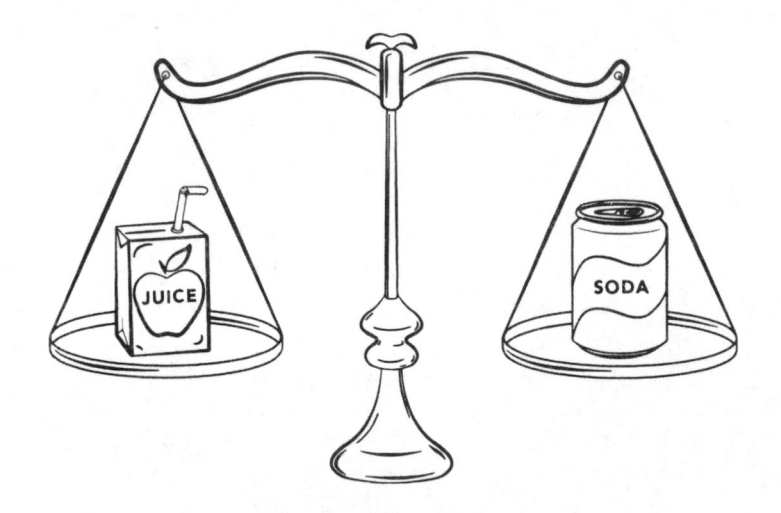

DRINK

The evil cousin of alcohol. While booze can have surprising health benefits, these "healthy drinks" somehow do the
opposite. Some of these, like fruit juice, are sneaky carri-
ers of sugar. Some are unhealthy in massive doses. And
some, like milk, have recently had their powers called into
doubt.

Diet Soda

The math seems pretty simple. Calories in, calories out. A regular Coke has 140 calories. Diet Coke has zero. This is why I switched to diet over a decade ago.

But what if diet soda is a Trojan horse, smuggling in evil properties that somehow make us fat?

The studies are mixed. (Aren't they always?) Some epidemiological studies indicate that diet soda helped people lose weight, some showed they gained weight, and some showed no difference. One study showed that diet soda was linked with a 67 percent higher risk of diabetes, another indicated that diet soda drinkers are 30 percent more likely to be depressed, and my own personal study indicates that men have a 5,000 percent higher chance of being laughed at when ordering Diet Coke on a date.

"Artificial sweeteners can contribute to excess weight gain, increased body fat, and diminished ability to regulate blood sugar levels," says Dr. Susan Swithers, a Purdue University researcher who, in 2013, tested the impact of artificial sweeteners in rats. Her findings triggered a flurry of headlines like "How Diet Soda Can Sabotage Your Diet" and "Study: Diet Soda Doesn't Help You Lose Weight."

There are at least two theories as to how diet soda could be fattening. The first is simple: people tell themselves that they're being healthy with Diet Coke, so now they eat more cookies as a reward. I don't find this particularly troubling. Yes, *maybe* it explains how

large-population studies show no weight loss with diet soda, but the dynamic is strictly psychological. It can be overcome with willpower. Skip the cookie and you'll be okay.

The second theory, though, is far more unsettling: diet sodas could change the way your body metabolizes sugar. Here's how it works: When you taste something sweet, your body gets a signal that it should prepare itself for the flood of incoming energy and sugar, so it releases hormones and ramps up the metabolism. But Swithers's research suggests that when you drink diet soda, your body is tricked into doing something else. When we use artificial sweeteners, "sweet tastes are no longer reliably followed by sugars and energy; the body then learns that it shouldn't produce these same kinds of responses because it can't anticipate what will happen," she tells me. "So when real sugars are consumed, the body can't anticipate that energy and sugars are going to show up, and it's less well prepared to deal with them."* Other research has reached similar conclusions.

In other words, Diet Coke is sort of like the Little Boy Who Cried Wolf. The artificial sugar warns your body to brace itself for higher glucose—but nothing happens. Then again nothing happens. Then again nothing happens. Finally, when the real wolf (sugar) actually shows up, the body no longer reacts as quickly, disrupting your metabolism.

So here's what I'm really curious about. Let's say you have to

---

*Not every scientist agrees. "The bloggers of the world have latched on to the notion that diet sodas cause obesity, but the science just isn't there to back it up," Dr. Barry Popkin, an obesity researcher at the University of North Carolina, tells WebMD.

choose between regular Coke and Diet Coke. Which one is better?

"It's just the wrong question to ask," Swithers responds. "No one should be drinking sodas of any kind every day."

Fair enough. But this is my (not very scientific) takeaway: with regular soda we *know* that it has sugars that boost our odds of getting fat. With diet soda it *might* have properties that boost our odds of getting fat. Would I be healthier ditching soda altogether? Probably. But that's not going to happen, so given the choice between two evils, I'll stick with the diet.

Water

One summer, every night before going to bed, I drank a canteen of water as fast as I could. When I finished, I would raise the canteen over my head, turn it over, and if a single drop spilled, I'd refill the canteen and guzzle a second.

I was in Marine Corps boot camp. The drill instructors yelled at us to "Drink, drink, drink! Drink, you maggots, drink!" So we drank. On the wall of every bathroom, a poster showed the optimal color of our urine: clear with just the wispiest trace of yellow.

The lesson stuck with me for life. It's been years since I wore a uniform or fired an M16, but I still pound the water and inspect my urine for clarity. It's the healthiest thing I do.

Only it might kill me.

"People are always surprised that you can drink yourself to death, but that's been well documented for over a decade," says Dr. Joseph Verbalis, a professor of medicine at Georgetown. In Sacramento, for example, a radio station held a contest—"Hold

Your Wee for a Wii"—promising a Nintendo to the person who chugged the most water before peeing. A woman drank 6 liters of water, felt sick, went home, and died. Similar water deaths have been caused by fraternity hazing. Right now you're probably thinking *Hey, but I'm not some knucklehead who wants to star on* Jackass. The same thought probably raced through the head of a British runner, aged twenty-two, who ran the 2007 London marathon, drank lots of water to stay hydrated, finished the race, then died. His profession? Fitness instructor.

Here's how it works: The average kidney can excrete about 20 liters a day. If you drink too much, too fast, the kidney falls behind and this leads to hyponatremia, an abnormally low blood level of sodium, an essential electrolyte. The water eventually makes its way to your brain cells, which, like rice, expand with water. But, unlike rice, brain cells are smushed up against your skull, so a swelling can trigger fun neurological issues like headaches, dizziness, a loss of consciousness, seizures, and strokes.

The wacky curveball: you are far more likely to die of hyponatremia when you think you need water the most. This is why marathon runners are especially at risk. When the body works harder, the kidneys are weakened and can only excrete 3 to 4 liters a day—about one-sixth of their at-rest efficiency. "Yes, you're sweating more and losing fluid, but by the same token you're not getting rid of everything you drink," says Verbalis, adding that in a study of Boston marathon runners, a staggering *14 percent* had symptoms of hyponatremia. "If you multiply that 14 percent by the hundreds of thousands of marathon runners each year . . ."

Gatorade won't really help, as Verbalis says the advertised "electrolytes" are a gimmick, and some of the deaths, in fact, happen to runners drinking Gatorade. How about munching on salty

snacks? "This might delay it, but it won't prevent it. The only way to prevent hyponatremia is to not drink too much water."

Okay, so what about my training with the Marines? Were they wrong?

"The U.S. Army realized that it was giving bad advice," he says. "It has since changed its guidelines for hydration."

Huh. What else have I been doing wrong?

The good news is that for most people, this isn't an issue. This is not a PSA to Stop Drinking Water. We need it. But the old saw "eight glasses of water a day" is a fairly arbitrary number, and "There's nothing backing it up," says Verbalis. "No evidence of any health benefit. There are only a very limited amount of people who need to drink that much water—like patients with kidney stones or some people with asthma."

But I need a rule! I need a maxim! I need to know—when should I drink water?!

"When you feel thirsty."

Even more bad news about water: Recent studies have shown that in countries like Bangladesh, Chile, and Taiwan, the public tap water could be laced with arsenic, and this arsenic could cause heart disease. In 2014, a professor from Johns Hopkins University showed that the same thing was possible in the United States. Whoa. Scary shit. Especially when you see something like this headline in the *New York Times*: "A Heart Risk in Drinking Water."

But what's the *absolute risk?* Should we be concerned? The story focuses on Native Americans who drink from private wells, and you have to read pretty closely to catch the detail, "Although the Environmental Protection Agency sets a 10 parts-per-billion safety standard for drinking water, only municipal water utilities are required to meet it." So, yes, if you live on a Native American

reservation or if you have a private well in your backyard, you should be worried. If you drink your water from a municipal water utility—99.9 percent of the readers of this book, 99.9 percent of the readers of the *Times*—then there's no need to freak out and buy bottled water. For some reason the *Times* didn't go with the more accurate headline: "Your Water Is Almost Certainly Safe, But Water from Private Wells—Which Only Represents Maybe 0.001 Percent of the Population—Might Have Heart Risk."

Fruit Juice

Drink 1: 165 calories, 39 grams of sugar
Drink 2: 140 calories, 40 grams of sugar

Drink 1 is apple juice. Drink 2 is a can of Coke. This information may cause cognitive dissonance, as we've been led to believe that apple juice is wholesome, righteous, American. It's something that Mom can give to little Timmy and then pat him on the head, wave good-bye, and watch him skip to Little League.

The problem is that when you liquefy fruit and dump it in a bottle, you lose its fiber, its flavor, and the chunks of fruit that make it fruit. What are you left with? Sugar. In 2014, British researchers at the University of Glasgow studied the health benefits (or lack thereof) of fruit juices, found them just as junky as sodas, and further cautioned that "current evidence suggests high fruit juice intake is associated with increased risk of diabetes." And yes, it's true they have scraps of micronutrients like vitamin C, but the researchers concluded that these "might not be sufficient to offset

the adverse metabolic consequences of excessive fruit juice consumption."

When you factor in human psychology, you could make the case that fruit juices are worse than soda, because we tend to think of them as healthy and therefore we drink them to excess. These clever Glasgow scientists tried to quantify just that. They conducted a survey of two thousand adults, showing them pictures of fruit juices and sodas, and asked them to guess how many teaspoons of sugar were in each one. People tended to underestimate the sugar in fruit juices by about 50 percent. We've tricked ourselves into drinking a "health drink" that is, essentially, just more soda. This is why I only drink whiskey.

Milk

Headline in *Forbes*: "Holy Cow! Study Suggests Milk Is Bad for Bones, Heart. Has the Medical Establishment Lied to Us?" (Bad pun, titillating results, and an accusation of mass malpractice, all in one headline. Well done, *Forbes!*)

The short version: In 2014, after tracking one hundred thousand Swedes for a period of over twenty years, researchers found a slightly higher mortality rate for women who guzzled lots of milk. And you know how milk is supposed to strengthen your bones? Maybe not. For women, at least, when they drank more milk, they actually had *more* hip fractures. (As *New York* mag put it, "Heroic Study Says Milk Is Bad for Women . . . Which Is Actually Solid News As Milk Is Revolting.")

So does this mean that milk is evil? Even the architects of this

study tell us not to freak out, saying, in typical researchery language, "Given the observational study designs with the inherent possibility of residual confounding and reverse causation phenomena, a cautious interpretation of the results is recommended." (Translation: correlation versus causation.) It's possible that other factors could explain the higher mortality rates, it's possible that people who were *already* at higher risk of hip fractures preemptively drank more milk, and it's possible that a sugar in milk, called galactose, does something weird to our bodies. It's hardly conclusive.

Most health experts seemed to have a similar reaction to the results: If you like drinking milk, continue drinking milk. If, however, you only drink it because you've been told it will strengthen your bones and help you live longer, well, quit wasting your time drinking milk.

Green Tea

Green tea is lauded for its health benefits. Often rightly so. Various studies suggest that it can do many wondrous things, including:

- Trim the risk of heart attack
- Lower the risk of Parkinson's
- Strengthen bones
- Unleash antioxidants that curb the risk of breast cancer, lung cancer, pancreatic cancer, and basically every kind of cancer
- Help people feel superior to coffee drinkers

In fact, green tea is one of those few drinks that, according to the experts, we're told we do *not* have to drink in moderation. The more the merrier. But not for a forty-seven-year-old woman who, in 2013, went to the hospital complaining of pain throughout her body. As the *Huffington Post* reports, her doctor "discovered that consuming 'astronomical amounts' of highly concentrated tea for nearly 20 years had caused her fluoride levels to spike to more than four times the normal amount." Her teeth became so brittle that they had to be yanked out.

To be fair, this isn't common. It makes for a catchy headline, but like many such headlines, there's very little absolute risk. According to the woman's doctor, "There have been about three to four cases reported in the U.S. associated with ingesting tea, especially large amounts of it."

The larger issue, though, is that plenty of stuff marketed as "green tea" is a far cry from the real McCoy. *Times* reporter Anahad O'Connor cited a recent analysis of commercial teas conducted by ConsumerLab.com, which found that "some bottled varieties appear to be little more than sugar water, containing little of the antioxidants that have given the beverage its good name." Some of the biggest culprits: Snapple Diet Green Tea had almost no traces of EGCG—*epigallocatechin gallate*, the substance that has all the antioxidant goodies. Green Tea with Honey, an Honest Tea brand, had only 60 percent of the catechins (antioxidants) it claimed. Many of the teas also contained traces of lead, but the researchers concluded the amounts were too small to be of concern.

Moral of the story: green tea is probably fine. But fake green tea is the nutritional equivalent of taking a fat man with a beard,

stuffing him into a red suit, and calling him Santa Claus. It's a placebo: it might trick the unsuspecting, but there are no real elves.

Breastfeeding

In ancient times, when new mothers used baby formula instead of the milk from their own breasts, they were stoned to death. Or at least it feels like that. The American Academy of Pediatrics recommends breast-feeding—and only breast-feeding—for the first six months. The Mayo Clinic warns, "The benefits of breast-feeding are well established. Consider ways to support breast feeding—and how to handle feelings of guilt if you can't or decide not to breast-feed." There's that word again: *guilt*. It's everywhere in the world of health. The message is clear as a bell: *If you wimp out and decide not to breast-feed, you are dooming your baby.*

So, what does the evidence say?

Traditionally, most studies have, in fact, shown a link between breast-feeding and the baby's health and wellness. But these observational studies are haunted by that old ghost of data analysis, the problem of correlation versus causation. Is it possible that women who choose to breast-feed tend to be more affluent, and maybe they have easier access to quality doctors, and they're more healthy to begin with?

In 2014, a researcher from Ohio State University tried to answer just that. As sociologist Cynthia Colen said at the time, the previous studies on the topic "either do not or cannot statistically control for factors such as race, age, family income, mother's employment—things we know that can affect both breast-feeding and health outcomes."

So her team looked at twenty-five years of data, and they measured the impact of breast-feeding on eleven variables of health such as obesity, hyperactivity, and body mass index. When they first crunched the numbers, sure enough, they did find the usual results from the usual epidemiologic studies—breast-feeding was linked with higher health. A win for the breast-feeders, right?

Not so fast. Then Colen's team took an inspired additional step: they filtered the results to look only at a smaller subset of the swamp of data—she looked at *pairs of siblings,* where one had been breast-fed, one bottle-fed. This controls for demographics. She had found a way to correct for selection bias. When she re-crunched the numbers, looking just at pairs of siblings, she found that in ten of the eleven categories, the benefits of breast-feeding practically vanished—they were no longer statistically significant. (Asthma was the sole exception.) "Our results suggest that typical estimates of the impact of breast-feeding on child wellbeing may be over-stated," she concluded.

Does this mean that we should stop breast-feeding and stock up on formula? Not necessarily. "I'm not saying breast-feeding is not beneficial, especially for boosting nutrition and immunity in newborns," said Colen. "But if we really want to improve mater-nal and child health in this country, let's also focus on things that can really do that in the long term—like subsidized day care, better maternity leave policies and more employment opportunities for low-income mothers that pay a living wage, for example." Trans-lation: Let's stop throwing stones.

Juice Cleanse

Here's the problem with juice cleanses:

1. It's a juice cleanse.
2. Yes, you will shed a few pounds, but the weight will almost certainly return when you start acting like a normal person again.
3. The entire "cleanse" premise, from a medical perspective, is sort of bullshit.

"Juice cleanses accomplish exactly none of their physiological or medical objectives; they fetishize a weird, obsessive relationship with food, and they are part of a social shift that reduces health (mental, physical, and, sure, spiritual) to a sign of status," argues Katy Waldman in *Slate*, concluding, "They're annoying as hell." No scientific studies have shown any long-term benefits.

This is the position of the Cleansers: Since our modern diets are heavy in trash like Fritos and Big Macs, the walls of our intestines are coated with layer upon layer of slime. Every day, every meal, we add more toxins to our gut. (Just what exactly is a toxin, you ask? As Waldman says, "After days of Googling I still have no idea WTF a toxin is. . . . The juicing industry is counting on that.") Since our innards are filled with these toxins, the logic goes, if we can give them a three- to five-day break—no intake of food— the body will have a chance to flush out the garbage. As the website BluePrintCleanse.com cheekily says on its Excavation option: "Hey paste eater! This option unearths those crayons and other art delicacies you chowed down on in third grade."

This does sound sort of logical. But as Dr. Liz Applegate, director of sports nutrition at UC Davis, tells me, "Your digestive system doesn't 'need a rest.' That's like saying your heart needs a rest." Your heart pumps blood. It's what it does. Your digestive system digests. It's what it does. The system doesn't need a weekend or a holiday. "A lot of laymen think that juicing will somehow strip you of items that get stuck in there. And that is absolutely not true."

Still, if it's good enough for Gwyneth Paltrow, how bad can it be? I decide to find out. To get the full cleansing experience, I opt for a DIY program that requires you to buy a juicer, "all-natural" herbal supplements, and what seems like 70 pounds of organic carrots. Here's the quick and condensed version.

Day 1

I start my day with the Breakfast of Champions: a "morning flush" of 24 ounces of warm water, spiked with lemon juice. It takes me a full hour to liquefy the apples and carrots, splattering my white counter with carrot juice that still, one year later, leaves an orange stain. The schedule requires me to drink every hour. I pour a dry mix called Bowel Formula #2 into one of my drinks; hours later I feel the consequences. I brew my "detox tea," which is a substitute for coffee the same way Kool-Aid is a substitute for beer.

Day 2

"Do you feel hungry?" everyone asks me. Oddly, not really. That's not the challenge. The larger, more practical issue is that you're beholden to a punishing schedule of juice-sipping. On a normal day for a normal person, if you're late to lunch it's no big

deal—you just eat later or you grab a snack. With a juice cleanse there are no mulligans. Your body limps along with *just* enough calories to fuel the engine, and if you miss one the system breaks down. There's no cushion. (This is oddly similar to my junk food cleanse.) Another practical issue: to carry these bottles of juice I lug around a small padded cooler, and it looks like, well, a fanny pack. The juice cleanse is not awesome for your dating life.

Day 3

My stool looks amazing. Like something out of a textbook. Sure, the whole cleaning-out-the-toxins thing might have been debunked by "scientists," and maybe it's psychosomatic, but my stomach does feel lighter, cleaner. And here's one surprising side effect of a juice cleanse: it gives you focus. It takes an extreme amount of attention to make sure you have the right drinks at the right times. I like it when my life has a little mission. Then again, it would also take focus to dig a twenty-foot hole in the Serengeti. This doesn't mean we should buy shovels and fly to Africa.

Day 4

A month ago I had scheduled a game of tennis. I think about canceling, as I barely have enough energy to read a book, much less swing a racquet. But I somehow bike ten miles and somehow play a match. I'm worried that I'll pass out without the benefit of food, but amazingly my energy levels are high. This, to me, is the true upside of juicing: It shows that your body is a remarkable thing. It's tougher than you think. You can starve it of calories and it can *still* function at a high level.

Day 5

Something curious happens: I *want more*. Maybe I could extend the cleanse to six, seven, or even ten days? Maybe I could set a juicing record. Reenergized on the way home from work, I buy more sacks of organic apples and organic carrots. Juicing now, juicing forever!

Hours later I come to my senses, and the next morning I gradually re-acclimatize myself with a bowl of cereal, then some fruit, and then a salad. Everything they promised was true: I no longer craved a burger, I wanted to change my diet, and in those five days alone I lost 6 pounds.

That was over a year ago. Since then I long ago added back the 6 pounds, I've eaten plenty of burgers, and my stomach is no doubt full of those "toxins." The benefits are fleeting. A juice cleanse isn't a healthy marriage; it's a one-night stand.

I don't regret doing the cleanse, but not because I think it's super healthy. It does have one real benefit: it's interruptive. It forces you to think about your diet, and it gives you a chance to reboot. Some of my friends use the cleanse as a way to kick-start a longer-term diet, and while that might have nothing to do with "toxins," they find it useful. I buy that.

Then again, the same thing can be done with Twix, Snickers, Nerds, and whiskey. The juice cleanse, just like almost every fad diet, is yet more proof that the laws of thermodynamics still apply: calories in, calories out. It's not magic.

Vitaminwater

INT. NEW YORK—OFFICE BUILDING—
ADVERTISING FIRM—DAY
Conference room. A team of advertising execs huddle around a table, brainstorming. Long meeting. They're frustrated. Don Dapper leads the meeting.

DON DAPPER: Okay people. We need a name for this shit. What do we have?

AD EXEC 1: Um . . . Sugar Water?

DAPPER: Are you high?

AD EXEC 2: But people like sugar . . .

DAPPER: You can't *call* it that. What else?

AD EXEC 2: Colored Water. It comes in blue, red, yellow—

DAPPER: Colored Water sounds like an Al Gore documentary. *Next.*

AD EXEC 3 (nervous): Um . . . Vitamin Water?

DAPPER: Now *that's* what I'm talking about. *(Pulls out a cigarette, lights it.)* Who else wants a vitamin stick?

And so Vitaminwater was born. It's proof that anything can be framed as a health benefit—even a bottle of water that's loaded with 13 grams of sugary carbs, about as many carbs as you'd find in a bottle of Guinness. Vitaminwater is basically soda. (The kicker? That's 13 grams *per serving,* and since the standard bottle has 2.5 servings, you're sucking down 35 grams of carbs, or more than a serving of Ben & Jerry's Chunky Monkey ice cream. In fairness, they do now offer a low-cal version.) My favorite bit of Vitamin-water trivia is that in 2009, Coca-Cola—Vitaminwater's parent company—was sued by a consumer advocacy group, which, on behalf of sane people everywhere, accused Coca-Cola of "deceptive labeling and marketing for the soft drink, which included claims that the drink could . . . promote healthy joints and support 'optimal immune function.'"

Coke's defense? The lawyers actually had the balls to argue—and I couldn't make this up—"No consumer could reasonably be misled into thinking Vitaminwater was a healthy beverage."

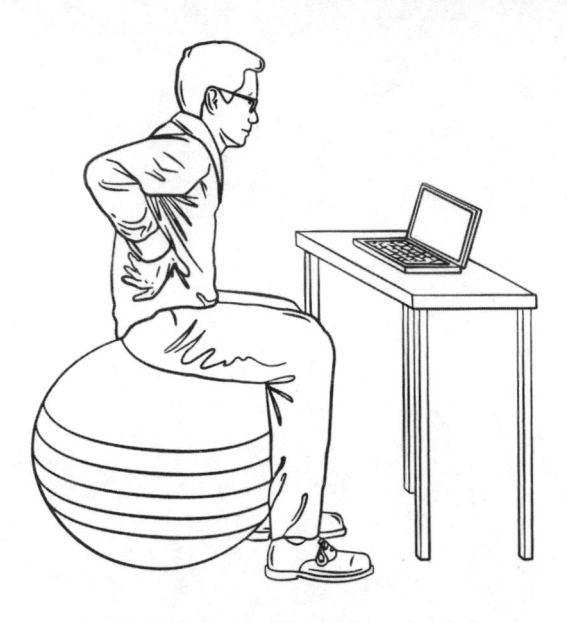

FITNESS

I believe that every human has a finite amount of heart-beats. I don't intend to waste any of mine running around doing exercises.—Neil Armstrong

The first time I see a jogger smiling, I'll consider it.—Joan Rivers

Standing Desks

The argument for stand-up desks is a powerful one: We spend too much of our lives sitting on our asses. We're a nation of sitters. Whereas our ancestors did awesome things like chase rabbits and beat each other with clubs, we plunk our butts at our desks, our cars, our sofas, our golf carts.

Gobs of research suggest that this sedentary lifestyle is responsible—or at least partly responsible—for the obesity epidemic. In an attempt to quantify our laziness, a telling (but tone-deaf) study found that in 1967, housewives spent 27 hours a week on active chores like cooking and vacuuming, but by 2010, this had plunged to 13.3. This burns roughly 360 fewer calories a day. It's an awkward study for a lot of reasons, and surely this also represents a positive trend toward women in the workplace, but still, we can infer that, in general, we're simply *doing less stuff* with our legs and arms. Another study compared men who were sedentary for 23 hours a week versus men who were sedentary for less than 11 hours a week, and found that the couch potatoes had a 64 percent higher chance of dying from heart attack. Even more sobering: The couch potatoes weren't actually couch potatoes but *also exercised regularly*. It turns out that exercise, by itself, isn't enough. We need more movement. I found this chilling. It's worth repeating: *even when we exercise, our sedentary nature is hurting us.*

Stand-up desks seem like an ingenious solution. After all, they

were used by Winston Churchill, and he's a paragon of health.* Only one problem: They're not any better. "Sitting all day is bad but so is standing all day! The key is a mix," says Dr. Alan Hedge, the director of Cornell's Human Factors and Ergonomics Research. "I recommend a pattern of 20 minutes sitting, 8 minutes standing and 2 minutes moving. It's really the moving that gives the greatest benefit because as muscles contract they help pump blood around the body."

When you use a stand-up desk, the first thing you notice is that you feel like a shmuck. You're *that guy*. The second thing you notice is that it's not any fun. Your feet hurt. Yes, it's true you don't feel as lazy, but it's also true that you don't feel the endorphins, energy, or enthusiasm you get from anything that resembles exercise. The standing desk is to staying active as Facebook is to staying in touch: It's not the real deal. (Others have had more success when they rigged a treadmill next to their desk; A. J. Jacobs, for example, wrote the majority of *Drop Dead Healthy* while walking at a steady 1 mph.)

Studies have pegged that standing requires, on average, 20 percent more energy than sitting. But any theoretical benefit is offset by the health risks, according to Hedge: "back pain, leg and feet discomfort, varicose veins, and some cardiovascular problems— the heart has to work harder when standing." It's also possible that when you tilt your computer upward, this can lead to wrist extension and carpal tunnel.

Hedge says he's not aware of any credible evidence showing the

---

*Other healthy Winston Churchill habits: sleeping in until 11:00 a.m., working from bed, and drinking Johnny Walker with breakfast. These are the perks you get when you rally the world to fight Hitler.

benefits of standing desks. Instead he stresses the need to increase *moving*. "Try organizing your work so that you can stand every 20 to 30 minutes. And use that time to make a phone call, walk to a printer, grab a coffee." It's this movement—not just the act of standing—that pumps blood through the muscles. (And it doesn't hurt that movement is free.)

I had intended to use the stand-up desk for a full month before making my verdict. Instead I used it for one morning, shut it down, then went outside to the fresh air and took a ride on my bike. *Yes*.

The stand-up desk is yet another illusory panacea. It's a gimmick solution to a more complicated problem.

Okay, so if they aren't the answer, what about another possibility—those iso-ball chairs?

Ball Chairs

It slices! It dices! It will cook your breakfast, save you money, help you lose 20 pounds, and give you an erection!

Those dorky iso-ball chairs are just one of the fifty thousand products that trick us into thinking that *Yes, I've found it. THIS is what I need to finally get in shape.* We're told by a friend or an infomercial or maybe even a personal trainer that if we swap our desk chair with an iso-ball, it will "engage our core" and give us abs like Channing Tatum.

Too bad they don't work.

"Dreadful," Hedge tells me. "They're okay for Pilates classes, but all the research studies show that they don't actually engage the core muscles when you are just sitting doing computer work. And there is a danger of falling off the ball and injuring yourself."

One such study was conducted by an expert of spine biomechanics and a professor at the University of Waterloo, Dr. Jack Callaghan, who instructed seven people to sit on normal chairs and seven people to sit on the bozo-chairs. Then he measured how these postures activated eight different core and back muscles. Conclusion? Nothing. Or, more precisely, the effect was so minuscule that it didn't offset the discomfort. Posture was not improved. There was no workout, no core-building, no Channing Tatum. Nothing but the awkwardness of sitting in a stupid chair.

"To be quite frank, I cannot see any advantage or reason for a person to be using an exercise ball as an office chair," Callaghan said at the time. Now, in fairness, another study did show that these bozo-chairs helped you burn 4 extra calories an hour. FOUR WHOLE CALORIES PER HOUR. If you work eight hours a day, this translates to a whopping total of 32 calories. That's less than one piece of bread.

Suggestion: Burn more calories with this hot new workout:

Step 1: Get a screwdriver. Either flathead or Phillips is fine.
Step 2: Stand next to your bozo-ball.
Step 3: Repeatedly strike the bozo-ball with the screwdriver until it is destroyed.

Stretching

Forget what you learned in gym class. Stretching is dead. Or, more accurately, *static* stretching before a workout has been shown—again and again, in study after study—to have no positive impact. Skip it.

"Static stretching tends to make you weaker," says Dr. Duane Knudson, a professor of kinesiology at Texas Tech University and the author of *Fundamentals of Biomechanics*. "It keeps you from activating your muscles as well as you could, and it makes you weaker for about thirty minutes to an hour."

Knudson was one of the earliest stretching skeptics, publishing the first controversial paper in 1998. At the time, this advice was so counterintuitive that people angrily wrote to the editor, saying he must be mistaken. He wasn't. "Now, after a hundred and fifty to two hundred research papers, maybe 80 percent of them conclusively show a negative effect of static stretching," he tells me. "The other small percentage shows no effect at all."

As just one of many examples, in a 2013 study from the *Journal of Strength and Conditioning Research*, scientists found that when a group of seventeen athletes did a barbell squat, their maximum rep was 8 percent lower when they stretched beforehand. Even worse? When they warmed up with static stretching, their lower-body stability declined by 23 percent. In a review of over one hundred studies, researchers at the University of Zagreb in found that, on average, static stretching makes our muscles weaker by 5.5 percent, and they're even weaker if we hold the pose for 90 seconds.

This is not to say that all stretching is evil. It's mostly a problem when it's static—what we were taught in gym class, basically—where we lace up our sneakers and then touch our toes. The body prefers a warm-up. "Tell your readers that stretching is okay to maintain normal amounts of flexibility, but you need to be warmed up beforehand. Warmer tissue is stronger and will absorb more energy before it breaks," says Knudson. So if you're going for a run, it's better to just start slow and gradually pick up steam. "There's

a subculture of distance runners who have qualitatively known this for fifteen, twenty years. They said, 'Stretching makes my legs feel bad' so they just gradually increased the intensity of their run."

This "bad news" struck me as enormously good news. I was delighted to trim a few minutes from my workouts, which allows more time to do healthy things like watch TV and eat ice cream.

Diets

So you're all excited about your new plan to lose 10 pounds? In the long term, according to the results of a 2014 meta analysis, and I'm paraphrasing here: *You're fucked.*

The analysis compared four different diets:

- Atkins
- Weight Watchers
- The Zone
- South Beach

The researchers combed through all the valid randomly controlled trials they could find, then aggregated the long-term results. Short version: Each diet basically did the same thing. As the researchers conclude (emphasis mine), "Our results suggest that all 4 diets are modestly efficacious at decreasing weight in the short-term, but that these benefits are *not sustained long-term*." Much of the weight came back in year 2. "While North Americans spend millions of dollars in the weight loss industry, available data are conflicting and insufficient to identify one popular diet as being more beneficial than the others."

"It basically says that all of the claims about one diet versus another diet—and everybody says they're the best—there's just no there there. There are no data to back it up. It's all diatribe," Katz said on *The Today Show*.* "As a culture we need to grow up about weight and health, and recognize they're like everything else. If you want to get there from here, it involves time, patience, and effort." Katz emphasizes the importance of a true *lifestyle* change and a desire to eat good, whole foods in sensible combinations.

Another longer-term study from 2007 found that while people tend to lose 6 percent of their body weight in the first year, that vanishes after year 5. The same study found that 41 percent of people tended to *gain more weight back* than they lost.

It's hard to see these results and not feel a touch nihilistic. Are we doomed? Should we just resign ourselves to a life of sloth, dreading the inevitable diabetes?

I have a different take. Yes, I agree with Katz that we need to embrace a more fundamental change to our lifestyle—not just use diets as a short-term fix—but I'm skeptical of test results that say "Diets don't work." It's true that maybe diets don't work long-term *on average*. But the "average" result doesn't apply to all people. In many studies, if you peer into the data, you see wild fluctuations with individual people; some might lose 20 pounds, some might lose none, some might gain 20. Success stories are lost in the noise of big data. Why do diets work for some people and not for others? Even though we spend $66 billion on the weight loss industry,

---

*I quote Katz a bunch not just because he seems like a good guy, but because he's *everywhere*. Every day he seems to write a new article on the *Huffington Post* or a new segment on a morning show. The man's a machine. Watch your back, Dr. Oz. . . .

there's still no consensus. So many variables are at play. Maybe it's genetic, maybe there are other environmental factors, maybe it's about willpower. I don't know.

But I do know that *for me*, and for plenty of others, it is absolutely possible to change the way that you approach food. It's possible to adopt better habits and make them stick. It's possible to eat in moderation and keep eating that way. The trick is to use the principles of a good diet—moderation—and then *keep practicing* until it's subconscious. When I needed to lose weight several years ago, for example, I tracked calories for two or three months. This is not fun. This is not sexy. This can get you laughed at in public. But once I tracked the calories and lost the weight I wanted to lose, I then had a deeply ingrained picture of what a moderate portion size looks like, and this informed my habits in the long-term. I'm not saying that this is the right strategy for everyone, but the fact that it did work for me, *long-term,* means I don't buy the notion that all diets are doomed.

The analogy is imperfect, but compare this to the economy. It's true that *on average* diets might disappoint in the long-term, just as it's true that *on average,* for most Americans, real wages haven't increased in thirty years. But the average masks the underlying details. The economy has plenty of economic winners and losers; some people get promotions, some people lose their jobs. We don't say, "Well, because the average income is staying roughly flat, I'm screwed and I'll never get a raise." We work harder, we work smarter, we try to separate ourselves from the pack.

Infomercial Fitness Products

Thigh masters. Gut busters. Tummy tucks. Ab rockers. Butt lifters. Compression shorts.

Worthless. All of them. At least that's what we can infer from a 2012 study by a team of Oxford researchers, who put a blow torch to the claims of fitness products. They reviewed 1,035 web pages, 100 general interest magazines, and 10 sports magazines to chronicle all the performance-enhancing claims, such as "Proven to quench thirst more effectively than water!"

What, exactly, does "Proven" mean? That's what the scientists wanted to find out. So they meticulously contacted the manufacturers of each and every one of the 100+ fitness products and performance-enhancing drinks that they saw advertised, asking for the details of their claims.

The conclusion? They were all bunk. "Half of all websites for these products provided no evidence for their claims, and of those that do, half of the evidence is not suitable for critical appraisal," wrote Dr. Carl Heneghan and the researchers. "No systematic reviews were found, and overall, the evidence base was judged to be at high risk of bias. Half of the trials were not randomised, and only 7 percent reported adequate allocation concealment."

"High risk of bias" is a polite way of saying that the company probably footed the bill for the study. In one case, when pressed, a protein manufacturer admitted that their "scientific evidence" was a 1930 study of rats. As the authors of the study note, "It is virtually impossible for the public to make informed choices about the benefits and harms of advertised sports products based on the

available evidence." And that's the problem. It's junk after junk after junk. "Most of them are a total waste of your money," Dr. Knudson (the professor of kinesiology) tells me. "I've had some colleagues who have tested things like the ab cruncher, and almost all of the studies show there's no difference from your traditional exercise. Save your money and just do one more regular push-up."

Okay, but what about the biggest health craze of the last twenty years, yoga?

Yoga

When type A men do yoga, they have a tendency to push themselves too far, too fast, which can result in broken ribs, twisted spines, and unfortunate attire.

William Broad is a Pulitzer Prize–winning science writer. He's also a lifelong yoga enthusiast. In his 2012 book *The Science of Yoga,* he sent a tizzy through the Land of Chakras by suggesting that, for some men, in some contexts, yoga does more harm than good.

"Yoga has produced waves of injuries. Take strokes, which arise when clogged vessels divert blood from the brain," writes Broad. "Doctors have found that certain poses can result in brain damage that turns practitioners into cripples with drooping eyelids and unresponsive limbs."

This is worth repeating: If you do yoga you will *turn into a cripple.* Okay, so maybe that's not entirely true. Broad admits it's a tiny percentage, and acknowledges that "the benefits unquestionably outweigh the risk." (The many benefits of yoga, of course, in-

clude lower stress, higher energy, improved flexibility, better sex, and the ability to live in Portland.)*

As for those wacky injuries, men do seem to be at higher levels of risk. "Guys who bend, stretch and contort their bodies are relatively few in number, perhaps one in five out of an estimated 20 million practitioners in the United States and 250 million around the globe," writes Broad. "But proportionally, they are reporting damage more frequently than women, and their doctors are diagnosing more serious injuries—strokes and fractures, dead nerves and shattered backs." Men are more likely to power through the pain, because we're dumb.

"Because the Americanized version of yoga is too often taught like an extreme sport, anyone with a current or past injury history shouldn't just jump into a yoga class," explains Dana Santas, a celebrity yoga trainer (for the NFL, MLB, etc.) in *Men's Health*. "Say you injured your right hip. While it was healing, another part of your body—such as your left knee—may have picked up the slack. Now, you walk into a yoga class where they do reclined hero's pose (where you're kneeling, but with your back on the floor). If your knee has already been stressed, the pose could cause your knee to pop because it puts the joint into extreme flexion. But how would you—or the instructor who has never met you before—know this?"

Broad also makes the point that while yoga *does* have a wealth of benefits that are legitimate, the Yoga Industrial Complex tends

---

*Loads of studies have linked yoga to lower mortality rates, fewer trips to the hospital, and lower odds of heart attacks. The absolute risk is low. The trade-offs are in its favor. Arguing that yoga (on balance) is a bad thing is like arguing that water is a bad thing.

to promote some iffy ones. Does yoga help burn calories? Maybe not. Yoga ain't easy, and the one time I tried Bikram yoga I was reminded of the punishments in Marine Corps boot camp, where you're forced to hold a rifle by your pinky for as long as you can. But certain branches of yoga are, by design, meant to be *slooooow-www,* and while this can be good for your body and mind, it might actually slow your metabolism.

"Yoga works so well at reducing the body's metabolic rate that—all things being equal—people who take up the practice will burn fewer calories, prompting them to gain weight and deposit new layers of fat," argues Broad. Of course, "all things being equal" is rarely the case, and it's possible—even probable—that when people take up yoga, they're nudged to be healthier in other ways: they eat better, they sleep better, they finally keep up with Oprah's Book Club. It's hard to swallow the idea that yoga makes you fat, but Broad argues that "when yoga succeeds at weight control, the scientific evidence suggests that it does so in spite of—not because of—its basic impact on the human metabolism." The science is also murky on whether yoga, at least in its traditional form, really counts as an aerobic exercise. Good for you? Yes. A replacement for running? Maybe not. (Hybrid classes like Yoga Boot Camp! are a different story.)

So the next time that pushy friend bugs you and says, "Oh my God you HAVE to come to yoga with me!" well . . . they're probably right. But at least now you have some counterarguments. Because who wants to be a cripple?

CrossFit

There's only one thing more exhausting than people who gush about how much they love CrossFit: people who complain about CrossFit. So we'll keep this short.

Yes, it gets people in shape. Yes, it's something of a cult. Yes, it can change your life. Exhibit A: my good friend Eric, who, in his late thirties, joined a CrossFit class and used it to build lean muscle, shed every ounce of fat, and whip himself into the best shape of his life (even better than high school, where he played on our football team. In *Texas*). He convinced his wife to join (she's now in great shape), then his son (ditto), and daughter (yep). They all love it. Their friends all love it.

The three knocks against it?

1. The injury risk. We've known about this for over a decade, when *The New York Times* ran a piece called "Getting Fit, Even If It Kills You." Then again, what high-intensity sport *doesn't* boost your risk of injury? Women gymnasts have a higher risk of tearing their ACLs: should we ban the trampoline? But CrossFit wears the risk of injury as a badge of honor. The founder and ringleader, Greg Glassman, once wrote, "We have a therapy for injuries at CrossFit called STFU."
2. Some argue that while CrossFit is an excellent way to get people off the couch and into the gym, the very nature of its "randomness" undercuts advanced training. Mark Rippetoe, the author of the weight-training bible *Starting*

Strength,* was affiliated with CrossFit for three years, teaching proper lifting technique. Then they parted ways. He acknowledges that CrossFit is "the greatest thing that has ever happened to barbell training, bar none, unequivocally and absolutely." But after people advanced past the novice stage, the program hits a dead end. "Once a person has adapted beyond the ability of random stress applied frequently under time constraints to cause further improvement, progress stalls. And increasing the intensity of the random stress doesn't work either—that just gets you hurt because you haven't gotten stronger, and your heart and lungs can only work at about 200 BPM and about 50 RPM," he writes in a *Huffington Post* op-ed. "CrossFit has an inherent problem that it cannot seem to solve."

3. It's the kale of weight lifting. *Enough* already, we get it.

Exercise

490 BC. The outmanned Greeks had just won a shocking upset against the Persians—some historians say it changed the course of Western civilization—at the battle of Marathon. A messenger named Pheidippides raced to Athens to share the incredible news. Legend says he ran over twenty miles. He didn't stop for breaks.

---

* *Starting Strength* is a great primer for anyone who wants to get serious about weight lifting. It's comically (and awesomely) meticulous. Most exercise books will devote a few paragraphs to explain how to do something like, say, a correct squat. For this one exercise, Rippetoe needs fifty-five pages.

He didn't drink Gatorade. He ran and ran and ran until he reached
Athens, he shouted the good news, and then, right there, he col-
lapsed. And died. The world's first marathoner died of a heart
attack. He wouldn't be the last.

Too much of anything is bad for you. Even exercise. Or as
the *Wall Street Journal* asks in a click-baity headline, "Is Endurance
Running the Exercise Equivalent of a Cheeseburger?" Multiple
studies have shown that while exercise tends to buttress cardiovascular health—plus the well-chronicled benefits of lowering
stress, boosting our metabolism, unleashing endorphins, trimming
the risk of diabetes and depression, yada yada—for endurance athletes, those benefits vanish at around thirty miles a week, and at
that point, the extra pounding can punish the heart.

I spoke with the indefatigable Gretchen Reynolds, the author
of *The First 20 Minutes*, and the writer of many of the fitness stories for the *New York Times* "Well Blog"—in other words, the person who knows more about fitness paradoxes than anyone on the
planet. "There is such a thing as too much," she tells me. "The evidence says there's a striking bell-shaped curve to exercise. Doing
nothing is very bad for you. And doing a whole, whole lot—at least
for some people—is bad for them. It's not just an increase of injury risk, but it may actually lead to a shorter life span." Echoing
the theme of this book, she says that it's a question of dosage—
and the right dosage appears to be, naturally, moderation.

Just a few of the counterintuitive findings:

- A 2014 British study found that in a group of roughly
  one thousand people with heart disease, over a ten-year
  period, the hard-chargers who exercised five or six days
  a week were more than twice as likely to die of a heart

attack than those who only exercised two to four days a week.

- Another study from the *European Heart Journal* examined cross-country skiers, finding a higher risk of heart arrhythmias (irregular heart beat) in the group that skied the longest and fastest.

- A 2013 study from the University of Montreal found that when they forced rats to train for a Rat Marathon—an hour a day for four straight months—their hearts were larger, which is good, but they also had scarring in the hearts, which is bad. (Whether this translates to humans is still unclear. But we do know for certain that if you are a rat, you shouldn't train for a marathon.)

- "Is Exercise Bad for Your Teeth?" asks *The New York Times* (written by Reynolds, as always). "Compared with the control group, the athletes showed significantly greater erosion of their tooth enamel. They also tended to have more cavities, with the risk increasing as an athlete's training time grew." The culprit wasn't Gatorade, as the researchers initially guessed, but rather the fact that when athletes really pushed themselves, their mouths produced less saliva, and saliva is useful for protecting teeth. (Am I the only one shocked that in light of this, Crest hasn't yet launched a Lebron James toothpaste? "Strong on the court. Strong on the teeth.")

- The most depressing of all: a 2014 study found that when people exercise, they tended to actually *gain weight;* the theory is that the workouts simply encouraged people to eat more. (Taubes makes this same point in *Why We Get Fat,* arguing that exercise is never a reliable way to lose

weight, as the more calories we burn, the more calories we eat.)

Doctor after doctor stresses that, in the big picture, exercise is still better than no exercise. "Exercise and even strenuous exercise is clearly associated with enormous heart health benefits in the vast majority of people when compared to people who do not exercise but, in a very small minority who have underlying problems, exercise can trigger arrhythmia," said Dr. Dermot Phelan, director of the Cleveland Clinic's Sports Cardiology Center. "While there is emerging evidence that prolonged strenuous exercise can increase risk of atrial fibrillation, the long-term risk of this is small compared to inactivity."

He's right to keep this in context. The sensational anecdote of someone dying in a marathon, for example, is not a rational reason to give up jogging. It might not even be a rational reason to give up marathons. Reynolds tells us that "even as participation in marathon racing almost doubled during the past decade, to more than 473,000 finishers in 2009 from about 299,000 in 2000, the death rate remained unchanged, and vanishingly small. A total of 28 people died during or in the 24 hours immediately after a marathon, most of them men, and primarily from heart problems. . . . Those numbers translate into less than one death per 100,000 racers." That super tiny risk of dying *while running a marathon* (less than 0.1 percent), according to cardiologist Dr. Paul Thompson, is more than offset by the assessment that "over all, running decreases the risk of heart disease." Translation: If you are thinking of running a marathon but worry that it's bad for your heart, this fear is misguided. (Once again, it comes back to the Perception Gap of risk.)

It's almost certainly better to jog a few miles than to sit on the couch, but what if those same three miles—which burn, say, 300 calories—seduce us into thinking that since we've paid our dues, we've now "earned" the next twenty hours of loafing? This explains how we gain weight. I've been guilty of this. In more weekends than I care to admit, I'd go for a quick morning jog and then, proud of this minor triumph, spend the next forty-eight hours watching football and gobbling nachos. The run itself isn't unhealthy. The mind-set is.

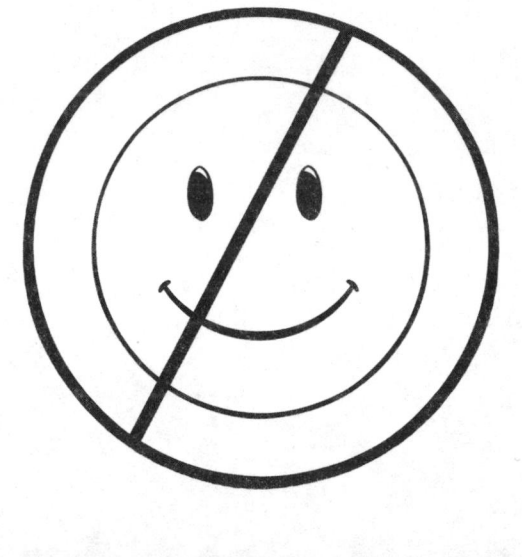

EVERYTHING ELSE

So now we're officially in "screwing around" territory. Use these topics to amuse your friends. Don't use these topics to change your life.

Marriage

Tons of studies have shown that stable, happy marriages are good for our health, or, to be more precise, good marriages tend to be "linked" with good health. (These are, of course, merely observational studies. To my knowledge, no one has ever taken a healthy group of twenty-somethings and forced group A to get married, group B to stay single, and then group C to take a sugar pill as a placebo.) The lead researcher of one study even felt so confident, he boasted, "It is as clear as day from the data that marriage, rather than money, is what keeps people alive." Over the years, scientists have proudly pointed to the health benefits of matrimony:

- Lower risks of dementia
- Lower overall mortality rates
- Less risk of cancer
- Healthier hearts
- Stronger bones
- Fewer car accidents
- Fewer hospital admissions
- More holiday cards sent and received

"I find the marriage/health link massively unfair. Nature is being a bit of a sadistic bastard," writes A. J. Jacobs in *Drop Dead Healthy*. "So you found your soul mate? Let's reward you with a long life

and freedom from sickness. Haven't been lucky enough to find that special someone? Sorry. You'll probably die sooner. It reminds me of how highly paid celebrities get free cars, shoes, and jewelry. Those of us without $15-million-per-movie contracts have to actually buy things."

The one tiny catch: not every marriage is a good marriage. And research suggests that if the union is wobbly, it cuts the other way. "The marriage advantage doesn't extend to those in troubled relationships, which can leave a person far less healthy than if he or she had never married at all," writes Tara Parker-Pope, author of *For Better: How the Surprising Science of Happy Couples Can Help Your Marriage Succeed.* "One recent study suggests that a stressful marriage can be as bad for the heart as a regular smoking habit. And despite years of research suggesting that single people have poorer health than those who marry, a major study released last year concluded that single people who have never married have better health than those who married and then divorced."

As always, it's tough to parse the correlation from the causation. It might just be that people who make rotten health choices also pick rotten spouses. Then again . . . researchers from Ohio State University demonstrated that when a couple has a domestic argument, the stress levels spike and the immune system suffers. Bickering takes a toll.

In one wickedly sadistic experiment, two groups of couples were given blisters on their forearms.*

---

*Remember the British doctor who, to measure the impact of profanity, asked volunteers to stick their hands in freezing water? I bet he'd like this one.

Couples from group A: just after the blisters, they were made to feel happy. (Researchers do this by asking them to talk about positive, supportive topics.)

Couples from group B: just after the blisters, they were made to bicker. (They were nudged to discuss topics of conflict.)

"The results were remarkable. After the blistering sessions in which couples argued, their wounds took, on average, a full day longer to heal than after the sessions in which the couples discussed something pleasant," explains Parker-Pope. "The study offered compelling evidence that a hostile fight with your husband or wife isn't just bad for your relationship. It can have a profound toll on your body."

This is a long-winded way of saying, "Mom, see, *this* is why I'm still single."

Two more things to note:

1. Happy marriages have also been correlated with weight gain. "On average, spouses who were most satisfied with their marriage were less likely to consider leaving their marriage, and they gained weight over time," said Dr. Andrea L. Meltzer, the lead researcher of a study from Southern Methodist University.
2. All relationships, by definition, end poorly: either in breakup or in death.

Choice

Imagine a horse. Now imagine that this horse is standing an equal distance between two bales of hay, and each bale of hay is exactly

the same size. The old parable says that this horse will die of hunger, as he is unable to make a choice.*

Too much choice can paralyze us. The good news is that if you are reading this book, you are not a horse. We all have the capacity to choose between more than two things. But as Dr. Barry Schwartz outlines in his book *The Paradox of Choice*, too much can be crippling. "When people have too much choice, they don't know how to choose, and they end up paralyzed," he tells me. "You go to a website and there are a hundred and fifty T-shirts, so you buy none. But if there are ten you might buy one."

This isn't just theoretical mumbo-jumbo. It has been extensively documented in both the worlds of psychology and marketing; the implications can cost a company billions. You can argue that one problem with the rollout of HealthCare.gov is that people were overwhelmed with all the choices, so some said, *screw it,* and then did nothing. In another context, Schwartz says that when states offered senior citizens fifty or sixty different medicines to choose from, they "made extremely sub-optimal decisions." They did better with only a handful of options.

When Steve Jobs returned to Apple from his mid-1990s exodus, he browsed through the catalog of products and flipped through the dozens and dozens of computers. So many. He ripped the manual to shreds and drew a simple 2 by 2 grid:

---

*(1) This parable comes from a paradox called "Buridan's ass," named after a fourteenth-century French philosopher, who originally conceived the idea as an ass who is equally hungry and thirsty, and he's standing exactly in between water and hay. (2) This has most definitely never actually happened.

	STANDARD	PRO
Laptop		
Desktop		

The Apple as we know it was born. This simplified both the company's operations and the consumer experience. Jobs reduced choice to keep it simple.*

Consider the case of online dating. It gives us thousands of options, but for some, this endless pool of possibility—Tinder, OKCupid, Match.com, *next! next! next! next!*—makes it tougher to make that one final decision. This effect has been quantified. In one 2011 study of speed-dating, for example, the researchers found that when people attended speed-dating sessions full of many people and therefore plenty of choice, they were less likely to *actually go on dates* than those who went to a smaller session with fewer choices.

The other problem with too much choice is that it boosts the odds of buyer's remorse. "Even if you overcome the paralysis and choose well, you might be dissatisfied," says Schwartz. "With so many options out there, it seems like there *had* to be a perfect option, and you missed it." In one of his studies, he compared two groups of college seniors looking for work:

1. Students who were "maximizers." They tended to exhaustively search all their options before making a decision.

---

*Of course this approach doesn't fly with everyone. The idea of Too Much Choice or Too Little Choice is the heart of the Apple versus Windows and Apple versus Android.

They indicated that for their job search, they would seek out and research many opportunities.

2. Students who were less rigorous about job selection.

Over the course of the next year, Schwartz and his team followed up on the kids, analyzed the outcomes (what kinds of jobs they landed), and gave them a battery of surveys that evaluated their psychological well-being. The results? The maximizers did land jobs that averaged 20 percent higher pay, but they *felt worse in every measured psychological category.* "We suggest that maximizers may be less satisfied . . . because their pursuit of the elusive 'best' induces them to consider a large number of possibilities, thereby increasing their potential for regret or anticipated regret, engendering unrealistic expectations, and creating mounting opportunity costs." (This is consistent with what we saw with happiness: an aggressive pursuit can backfire.)

As always, of course, the dosage matters. Too little choice can be even worse. Just consider the other end of the dating-choice spectrum: arranged marriages.

News

The news is chronically bad. We consume a ton of news. And yet there's very little discussion about how this exposure to rotten news—from TVs to our phones to our Apple Watches—impacts our health. "News is toxic to your body," argues Rolf Dobelli in a column for the *Guardian.* "It constantly triggers the limbic system. Panicky stories spur the release of cascades of glucocorticoid (cortisol). This deregulates your immune system and inhibits the

release of growth hormones." He compares news to sugar: we crave it, we get a rush from it, and then we want more of it. Yet somehow it leaves us hungry.

Blood and death aren't new phenomena, but our ability to see them is. Can you imagine CNN and Twitter during the Civil War? #BrotherOnBrother. This takes a toll. In the wake of the Boston marathon bombings, for example, researchers from UC Irvine tried to measure the impact of sensationalist news coverage. "People who exposed themselves to six or more hours of media daily actually reported more acute stress symptoms than did people who were directly exposed—meaning they were at the site of the bombings," researcher Alison Holman told NPR. Let's repeat that. *People exposed to the news reported just as much stress as people at the bombings.**

You could make the argument that when the news is consumed in snack-size nuggets, not only is it stressful, it's actually counterproductive. It just fuels our ADD and prevents deeper thinking. (Think of the difference between watching two minutes of GMA and reading *The Economist* cover to cover.) "The more news we consume, the more we exercise the neural circuits devoted to skimming and multitasking while ignoring those used for reading deeply and thinking with profound focus," Dobelli gloomily argues. "Most news consumers—even if they used to be avid book readers—have lost the ability to absorb lengthy articles or books."

I'm not sure I totally buy that, just like I don't believe that *all sugar* is bad or that we should never consume it. Tawdry news has

---

*One media study found that there are seventeen negative news stories for every one positive. Welcome to Newsroom 101: "If it bleeds, it leads."

its place. Maybe ignorance is bliss, but I'm sure somewhere there's bad news about bliss, and this news will make us stressed, but that's okay because stress can be a good thing, but hopefully not too much of a good thing because happiness can be bad for us, but that's okay because failure can be positive, but hopefully not so positive that we can retire early, because early retirement can be unhealthy.

College Degrees

There's nothing bad about college degrees . . . if they're free. But they're not. Since 1983, the average cost of a college diploma has not doubled, not tripled, but nearly *quintupled*, soaring past the rate of inflation. Salaries aren't keeping pace. The debt is choking. You can make the case that for some students—*some* students, certainly not all, and probably not most—plunking down $200,000 is an "investment" that has no chance of paying out.

It's an issue that's only barely in the scope of this book, so we'll keep this brief. Yet it shows how the same principles we see with food, fitness, habits, and attitudes also apply to things like financial investments and serious life choices—everything has a trade-off. Often we fail to fully analyze that trade-off.

"There is no simple answer to the question 'Is college worth it?' Some degrees pay for themselves; others don't. American school kids pondering whether to take on huge student loans are constantly told that college is the gateway to the middle class," reason the cooler heads at *The Economist*. "The truth is more nuanced, as Barack Obama hinted when he said . . . 'folks can make a lot more' by learning a trade 'than they might with an art history de-

gree.' An angry art history professor forced him to apologize, but he was right."

Should mailmen invest in a bachelor's degree? Should we encourage a mechanic to rack up $90,000 in student loans that might drive him to bankruptcy? What if he instead spent that $90,000 on a down payment for a house?

The issue is complicated. It forces us to ask uncomfortable questions about basic fairness (are we giving up on kids too early?), discrimination (is there a class or racial bias here?), and values (even if a college degree doesn't make *economic* sense, shouldn't the mechanic experience the joys of Proust?). Think-tankers seem to agree that for *most* students, you need a college degree more than ever before. It's essential. As Andreas Schleicher, the education directorate of the Organization for Economic Cooperation and Development, said in 2013, "Probably in these times there is no better investment you can make than in your education. Rate of return is in the order of 10 to 15 percent."

Enough with this downer topic. Next up, let's look at something absolutely ridiculous.

Height

If you are too tall, you will die.

Okay, that's not quite accurate. (Although in one sense it's 100 percent accurate, as you will die, eventually, whether you are too tall or too short.) The point is that there's no reason to have a Napoleon complex, as research suggests a correlation between height and a risk of dying younger.

On the surface this makes no sense, as we have long associated

height with both success (see: George Washington) and sex appeal (see: Dikembe Mutombo). For thousands of years we've been growing taller and living longer, so surely one is linked with the other, right?

But researchers from the Albert Einstein College of Medicine found something startling: in a 2013 study of 20,928 postmenopausal women, they found that when women are taller, they're more likely to get cancer. Specifically, every additional 4 inches of height boosts the odds of cancer by 13 percent.

So does height cause cancer? No. It can, however, be an indicator of increased growth hormones, and hormones *can* swing the odds of cancer. "We know that cancer is a disease in which hormones and growth factors modify things," said Dr. Geoffrey C. Kabat, chief researcher of the study. "Height itself is not a risk factor, but it really appears to be a marker for one or more exposures that influence cancer risk."

Being taller means that you have more bits of flesh and bones and muscles, and all of these pesky things can cause problems. This could be the reason that a 2012 study of Sardinian soldiers found that men who were five-foot-three or shorter tended to live an extra two years. "The fact that tall people die younger appears to be an immutable physical reality," *Slate*'s Brian Palmer explains. "A short person is like a Honda Civic: compact and efficient. Tall people are Cadillac Escalades. With all that extra weight and machinery, something's just bound to go wrong."

As you are sick of hearing, it's nearly impossible to split the correlation from causation. (So parents, don't starve your kids in the hopes that they will stay short and live longer.) But we can make some inferences. Maybe it's not shocking that Yao Ming, for example, had to retire early because his seven-foot, six-inch frame

put too much stress on his feet. Or take the midge, an insect that often bites people in the forests of Scotland. Scientists tracked the midge and somehow found that these insects are far more likely to bite tall people. "The preference for taller people could be associated with midge behavior and flight patterns, as midges are found at great numbers with increasing height, particularly between 1–4 meters," suggested researcher Dr. James Logan.

But that's all just anecdotal. If we want a more rigorous scientific study, look no further than the giant bald Nazi who fought Indy in *Raiders of the Lost Ark*, who had his head chopped off by the plane's propellers. Height kills.

Retirement

Behind on your 401(k) contributions? Good news! You could be dodging a bullet.

We think of retirement as the golden reward for a lifetime of diligence, but studies have shown that retirement itself—even controlling for age—is linked to higher risks of depression, divorce, strokes, and heart attacks. According to the American Institute of Stress, retirement is ranked as number ten on the list of life's most stressful events. (Things more stressful than retirement: death of a spouse, losing your job, imprisonment, and somehow both divorce *and* marriage. Things less stressful than retirement: death of a close friend, switching jobs, sexual difficulties.)

This is actually a pretty big social problem. There are about a hundred thousand people a day becoming eligible for Social Security, and that's expected to continue for the next twenty years. A few unsettling facts:

- The average retirement age is only sixty-two to sixty-three.
- Life expectancy is now seventy-nine.
- Only 13 percent of retirees are confident they've saved enough money.
- Two-thirds of retirees have saved *less than one year's salary.*

Retirees are 40 percent more likely to have a heart attack than nonretirees of the same age, according to a 2012 study from Harvard. These results are consistent with a 2013 British study, "Work Longer, Live Healthier," which found that retirement increases the risk of clinical depression by 40 percent. (The authors acknowledge that these types of studies are "inherently difficult because of the fact that, just as retirement can influence health, health can influence retirement decisions.")

Robert Delamontagne ran a company for twenty-five years, and when it was sold to Kaplan, he retired at age sixty-three. He stops short of calling his emotional state depression, but he knew something was wrong, so he researched. "The psychological adjustment to retirement is a dirty little secret," he tells me. "People don't like to talk about it because it's embarrassing." Instead of staying retired, Delamontagne hatched a second career with the book *The Retiring Mind*. So, what are the health risks of retirement?

"I'll give you the Top 10," he tells me. His list:

1. Reduction of intellectual stimulation.
2. Reduction of social stimulation.
3. Reduced feeling of contributing to a team.

4. Diffused sense of identity. (Especially for people who are high achievers. Delamontagne says, "The people who are the movers and shakers, the hard-chargers, the high-energy guys—when they retire, most of them have no idea what to do." The slackers tend to have an easier time in retirement.

5. Altered template for marriage. "A lot of people who are married have personality conflicts built into the nature of their relationships," and when they're working, it's easy to sweep those under the rug. "But when people are thrown together 24/7, they can become irritated and aggravated just because of the sheer amount of time they spend together." In most age ranges across the country, the divorce rate is actually *declining* . . . except for people over the age of fifty-five. Fifteen years ago, in that age bracket the divorce rate was 10 percent; now it's 25 percent.

6. All the time in the world with no idea how to fill it.

7. Threats to self-esteem. (There's no one to impress with, "*Do you know who I am?!? I'm the CEO!*" But you're no longer the CEO. You're just an old man at a diner who wants more toast.)

8. Shift from active to passive lifestyle.

9. Increased need for time management. Not so much in the day-to-day (they have plenty of that), but in terms of how to fill the remaining years . . . especially when you don't know how many there are.

10. Greater dependency on investment decisions. When you're twenty-three you can put all your 401(k) chips in the stock market, knowing you have thirty-plus years for it to yo-yo up and down. When you need that income

in twelve months? Suddenly you're watching CNBC like your life depends on it—which, in some ways, it does.

This is why, according to my financial forecasting, I'm on track with retiring at age 179.

Moderation

A little joke. But with a little bit of truth. A growing body of research suggests that in the case of exercise, if the objective is to burn fat, then short bursts of energy are more effective than our little prince: moderation.

Welcome to the era of high-intensity interval training, or HIIT. As a trainer once instructed me, "Get on the treadmill, slowly jog for two minutes, crank up the speed, go as fast as you can for one minute, then slow it down for two minutes, then a one-minute sprint, then a two-minute jog, then a one-minute sprint, and then you're done." This entire workout takes nine minutes. Multiple studies have shown that this burns more fat than thirty minutes of moderate exercise—specifically more abdominal fat. There's also evidence that these agonizing, *Rocky*-montage sessions of HIIT are better than moderate exercise at boosting endurance, lowering blood pressure, and lowering insulin resistance.

"The magic of high-intensity interval training lies in its ability to keep you burning fat even after you leave the gym," explains *Men's Fitness* trainer and writer Jeremy DuVall. "In short, your body isn't able to bring in enough oxygen during periods of hard work. Therefore, you accumulate a 'debt' of oxygen that must be repaid post-workout in order to get back to normal. The result: your me-

tabolism is revved for hours after you leave the gym. Trainers refer to this phenomena as excess post-exercise oxygen consumption, or EPOC." It's painful but it works.

Laughter

In the most joyless study of all time, in 2013, a team of British researchers decided to chronicle the many health risks of laughter. Sadly, this was not a clinical study where one group of people was induced to laugh and a control group was forced to watch *Two and a Half Men*. Instead, these grumpy bastards combed through 785 other studies that involved laughter, cherry-picking the ones that show a detrimental effect. At least the scientists had a sense of humor about it, calling their paper "Laughter and MIRTH (Methodical Investigation of Risibility, Therapeutic and Harmful)."

They first acknowledged that laughter has many proven health benefits, including:

- Reduced anger
- Reduced anxiety
- Lower risk of depression
- Lower risk of stress
- Reduced tension (psychological and cardiovascular)
- Increased pain threshold
- Improved lung function
- Reduced blood glucose concentration

Then they note that excessive laughter has been found to cause fainting, lead to asthma attacks, give you a headache, dislocate

your jaw—and in certain very rare instances, too much laughter can rip a hole in your esophagus. "Laughter is not purely beneficial. The harms it can cause are immediate and dose-related, the risks being highest for Homeric (uncontrollable) laughter," write the coauthors, Dr. Robin E. Ferner and Jeffrey K. Aronson. Happily, they conclude, "The benefit-harm balance is probably favourable. It remains to be seen whether sick jokes make you ill or jokes in bad taste cause dysgeusia, and whether our views on comedians stand up to further scrutiny."

It should be noted that while the study was indeed peer-reviewed, it appeared in the *British Medical Journal's* annual Christmas issue, which tends to skew tongue-and-cheek. "We don't know how much laughter is safe," Ferner said at the time. Then, slyly satirizing the cliché that you'll now find quite familiar, he added, "There's probably a U-shaped curve: laughter is good for you, but enormous amounts are bad, perhaps."

Just to be safe, since laughter can indeed be bad for you, I've gone through the book and edited out all the good jokes.

Final Thoughts

There's one final dynamic we should quickly explore. It's a health problem called *orthorexia.* This is so shamelessly self-serving that it sounds fake, but it's a real condition where people become so obsessed with health—so choosey about their foods—that they're nearly paralyzed. Eating pure is *hard*. For those stricken with orthorexia, the unrelenting battle of seeking grass-fed, non-GMO, pesticide-free food tends to cause stress.

"Some doctors and registered dietitians say they are increasingly

seeing people whose desire to eat pure or 'clean' food—from raw vegans to those who cut out multiple major food sources such as gluten, dairy and sugar—becomes an all-consuming obsession and leads to ill health," reports Sumathi Reddy in *The Wall Street Journal.* "In extreme cases, people will end up becoming malnourished." It's the health-nut cousin of anorexia. As one psychologist said, "It's just sort of a mind-set where it gets taken to an extreme like what we see with other kinds of mental illness." Doctors are working on treatment options as we speak.

How common is it? Dr. Thomas Dunn, a psychologist at the University of Northern Colorado, was one of the first to research orthorexia. "We don't know how prevalent it is. There's no data," he tells me. "But there are a lot of people walking around with it who are 'sub-clinical.' And their psychologist doesn't treat them. Their primary care doctor doesn't treat them." This can even trickle down to the children. Just as teenagers might feel an unhealthy pressure to be skinny, in some households, kids feel the pressure to eat pure. "We're seeing a lot of anxiety in these kids," the director of the eating disorders program at the University of North Carolina at Chapel Hill, Cynthia Bulik, told *The New York Times.* "They go to birthday parties, and if it's not a granola cake they feel like they can't eat it. The culture has led both them and their parents to take the public health messages to an extreme."

That last word is key: *extreme.* If you take away nothing else from this book, remember that the extremes, in nearly every facet of health, are dangerous. Too much dosage kills. This is even true of water, soy, kale, and yoga. Extreme diets don't work in the long run. Extreme marathons can be bad for your heart. An aggressive "pursuit of happiness" can make us less happy.

The ultimate irony, of course, is that the entire basis of

orthorexia—the glorification of organic, the vilification of BPA—isn't quite rooted in science. Or, to be more charitable, some studies agree with the purists; many others do not. The waters are muddy. Instead, Dunn suspects that orthorexia is rooted in *fear*. "It might come from an evolutionary drive to avoid poison, to avoid things that are disgusting. But this is taken to an extreme." (Earlier in the book we saw that disgust can have merit—now we see that it can go too far.)

So if you're a super healthy person and you do all the super healthy stuff—you run marathons, you grow all your own food, you never touch gluten—excellent, keep on being super. But for the other 99 percent of us, let's cut ourselves a little slack. We're probably better off not sweating the small stuff. If you feel inadequate because Marathon Joe is using a stand-up desk, well, now you know the joke's on him. That dude at the basketball court who touches his toes for five minutes, well, he's just weakening his muscles. So you drink boring old tap water instead of Vitaminwater? Good call. You're exercising four times a week instead of the six you promised yourself? You might be better off. You forgot to use Q-tips? Good, never use them again. You eat only candy bars instead of vegetables? Well . . . you're on your own. The basics still matter.

One final paradox: health has more nuance than we get from the headlines, but somehow, at the same time, it's simpler. The nuance: each study must be considered in the context of dosage, trade-offs, and relative versus absolute risk. The simplicity: once we use that framework, we're less exasperated by the herky-jerky nature of the news. It all begins to make sense.

You already know what you need to be healthy. There's no need to get distracted by the Flavors of the Month or the Demons of

the Month. Fat was never that bad. And kale was never that good. Both have their place.

One final thing that's bad for you: Books that are too long. So let's end this sucker now to keep the page count, like all else, in moderation.

Sources

INTERVIEWS

The following were interviewed by telephone, e-mail, or in person:

Alan Hedge, by telephone, July 29, 2014

Allan Brett, by telephone, August 14, 2014

Andrew Newberg, by telephone, July 24, 2014

Barry Schwartz, by telephone, August 19, 2014

Brett Ford, by e-mail, August 22, 2014

Carol Goman, by e-mail, July 28, 2014

David Allison, by telephone, September 9, 2014

David Katz, by telephone, June 4, 2014

David Tovey, by telephone, October 28, 2014

Denise Pope, by telephone, July 25, 2014

Donald Marcus, by telephone, August 26, 2014

Duane Knudson, by telephone, July 24, 2014

Gloria Mark, by e-mail, August 4, 2014

Gretchen Reynolds, by telephone, November 14, 2014

Ivan Oransky, by telephone, April 29, 2015

John Norcross, by telephone, October 8, 2014

Joseph Verbalis, by telephone, April 14, 2014

Karina Schumann, by e-mail, July 29, 2014

Katherine Beals, by e-mail, June 25, 2014

Liz Applegate, by telephone, May 7, 2013

Nancy Rojas, by e-mail, August 29, 2014

Nina Teicholz, by telephone, September 4, 2014.

Robert Delamontagne, by telephone, June 10, 2014

Robert London, by telephone, April 21, 2014

Rochelle Bilow, by e-mail, February 13, 2015

Steven Salzberg, by telephone, April 17, 2014

Stuart Lewis, in person, September 22, 2014

Susan Swithers, by telephone, August 15, 2014

Thomas Dunn, by telephone, March 13, 2015

FOOD
Kale

Jennifer Berman, "Kale? Juicing? Trouble Ahead," *New York Times*, January 1, 2014.

Lecia Bushak, "The Dark Side of Broccoli and Kale: Could Cruciferous Vegetables Be Bad for You?" *Medical Daily*, January 24, 2014.

Maria Godoy and Eliza Barclay, "Is It Time to Cool It on Kale Already?" NPR, October 2, 2013. www.npr.org/blogs/thesalt/2013/10/02/228499704/is-it-time-to-cool-it-on-kale-already

Drew Grant, "Can Kale Kill You?" *New York Observer*, January 14, 2014.

"Stars Who Love Kale," *US Weekly*, www.usmagazine.com/celebrity-body/pictures/stars-who-love-kale-2013238/32326, accessed July 15, 2014.

Low Fat

Kerry Torrens, "The Truth About Low-Fat Foods," BBCGoodFood.com, accessed August 27, 2014. www.bbcgoodfood.com/howto/guide/truth-about-low-fat-foods

Allison Aubrey, "Cutting Back on Carbs, Not Fat, May Lead to More Weight Loss," *NPR*, September 1, 2014. www.npr.org/blogs/thesalt/2014/09/01/344315405/cutting-back-on-carbs-not-fat-may-lead-to-more-weight-loss

"Fats and Cholesterol: Out with the Bad, in with the Good," *The Nutrition*

Source, Harvard School of Public Health, accessed November 15, 2014. www
.hsph.harvard.edu/nutritionsource/fats-full-story/

Gary Taubes, *Why We Get Fat: and What to Do About It*, Anchor, 2011.

Kathleen Zelman, "Low-Fat Diet: Why Fat-Free Isn't Trouble-Free," WebMD
.com, October 2, 2014. www.webmd.com/diet/low-fat-diet

Breakfast

Joan Salge Blake, "To Lose Weight: Eat Breakfast Like a King, Dinner Like a
Pauper," *Boston.com*, August 12, 2013. www.boston.com/lifestyle/health
/blog/nutrition/2013/08/to_lose_weight_eat_breakfast_l.html

"Eating a Big Breakfast Fights Obesity and Disease," ScienceDaily.com, August
5, 2013. www.sciencedaily.com/releases/2013/08/130805131011.htm

D. Jakubowicz et al., "High Caloric Intake at Breakfast Versus Dinner Differen-
tially Influences Weight Loss of Overweight and Obese Women," *Obesity*,
December 2013: 2504–12, doi: 10.1002/Oby.20460.

Gretchen Reynolds, "Is Breakfast Overrated?" *New York Times*, August 21, 2014.

Soy

Lindsey Konkel, "Could Eating Too Much Soy Be Bad for You?" *Scientific American*, November 3, 2009.

Frozen Yogurt

Hugh Merwin, "Fro-No: How New York City Soured on Frozen Yogurt,"
GrubStreet.com, May 15, 2014. www.grubstreet.com/2014/05/new-york
-city-frozen-yogurt-boom-is-over.html

Nutritional information found on Pinkberry.com.

Fish

Jane Brody, "Lots of Reasons to Eat Fish," *New York Times*, August 18, 2014.

"Fish: Friend or Foe?" *The Nutrition Source*, Harvard School of Public Health,
accessed October 1, 2014. www.hsph.harvard.edu/nutritionsource/fish/

Mary Anne Hansan, "Open Letter to Journalists," AboutSeafood.com, accessed
October 6, 2014. https://www.aboutseafood.com/press/open-letter-journalists

"Higher Blood Omega-3s Associated with Lower Risk of Premature Death
Among Older Adults," Press release, Harvard School of Public Health, April
1, 2013.

"Mercury in Fish More Dangerous Than Believed; Scientists Urge for Effective Treaty Ahead of UN Talks (Report)," *Huffington Post*, December 4, 2012. www.huffingtonpost.com/2012/12/04/mercury-in-fish-study-more-dangerous-treaty-un-talks_n_2238923.html

Laura Griesbauer, "Methylmercury Contamination in Fish," CSA—Discovery Guides, accessed October 6, 2014.

David Ropeik, *How Risky Is It, Really? Why Our Fears Don't Always Match the Facts*, McGraw-Hill, 2012.

"Superfish: A Warning to Seafood Lovers," PBS.com, July 15, 2009. www.pbs.org/wnet/nature/superfish-a-warning-to-seafood-lovers/1008/

Smoothies

Nutritional information from McDonalds.com. www.mcdonalds.com/us/en/food/full_menu/desserts_and_shakes.html

Nuts

Tim Ferriss, *The 4-Hour Body: An Uncommon Guide to Rapid Fat-Loss, Incredible Sex, and Becoming Superhuman*, Harmony, 2010.

James Hamblin, "The Dark Side of Almond Use," *Atlantic*, August 28, 2014.

Salad

Nicholas Bakalar, "Leafy Vegetables Often Cause Food Poisoning," *New York Times*, February 4, 2013.

"CDC: Leafy Greens Most Common Culprit Behind Food Poisoning," CBSNews.com, January 29, 2013. www.cbsnews.com/news/cdc-leafy-greens-most-common-culprit-behind-food-poisoning/

John A. Painter et al., "Attribution of Foodborne Illnesses, Hospitalizations, and Deaths to Food Commodities by Using Outbreak Data, United States," nc.cdc.gov, March 2013, doi: 10.3201/eid1903.111866

Michael Pollan, *The Omnivore's Dilemma: A Natural History of Four Meals*, Penguin, 2007.

David Zinczenko, "20 Salads Worse than a Whopper," MensHealth.com, accessed October 27, 2014. http://my.menshealth.com/exclusive-content/20-salads-worse-whopper?page=0,1

Margarine

"Fats and Cholesterol: Out with the Bad, in with the Good," *The Nutrition Source*, Harvard School of Public Health, accessed November 15, 2014. www
.hsph.harvard.edu/nutritionsource/fats-full-story/

Fruit

Sophie Egan, "Making the Case for Eating Fruit," *New York Times*, July 31, 2013.

David Katz, "Fructose, Fruit, and Frittering," LinkedIn.com, August 2, 2013. https://www.linkedin.com/pulse/20130802120959-23027997-fructose
-fruit-and-frittering

Gary Taubes, *Why We Get Fat: and What to Do About It*, Anchor, 2011.

Abigail Zuger, "A Diet Manifesto: Drop the Apple and Walk Away," *New York Times*, December 27, 2010.

Organic Food

Allison Aubrey, "Are Organic Tomatoes Better?" NPR, May 29, 2008. www.npr
.org/templates/story/story.php?storyId=90914182

Mark Bittman, "That Flawed Stanford Study," *New York Times*, October 2, 2012.

Kenneth Chang, "Stanford Scientists Cast Doubt on Advantages of Organic Meat and Produce," *New York Times*, September 3, 2012.

Tamar Haspel, "Is Organic Better for Your Health? A Look at Milk, Meat, Eggs, Produce and Fish," *Washington Post*, April 7, 2014.

Jennifer Welsh, "Is Organic Food All It's Cracked Up to Be?" *Business Insider*, May 13, 2013.

Christie Wilcox, "Are Lower Pesticide Residues a Good Reason to Buy Organic? Probably Not," *Scientific American*, September 24, 2012.

HABITS
Homework

Katy McLaughlin, "Pencils Down: Stop the Homework Insanity," *Wall Street Journal*, September 9, 2012.

Kamala Nair, "Too Much Homework: Bad for Kids?" Parenting.com, accessed July 28, 2014. www.parenting.com/article/too-much-homework-bad-for
-kids

Clifton Parker, "Stanford Research Shows Pitfalls of Homework," Stanford.edu, March 10, 2014. http://news.stanford.edu/news/2014/march/too-much -homework-031014.html

Natalie Wolchover, "Too Much Homework Can Lower Test Scores, Research- ers Say," *Huffington Post*, March 31, 2012. www.huffingtonpost.com/2012 /03/30/too-much-homework-test-scores_n_1391134.html

Holly Yettick, "Study Finds High School Homework Helps, Harms Students in Affluent Communities," Blogs.EdWeek.org, March 12, 2014. http://blogs .edweek.org/edweek/inside-school-research/2014/03/homework.html

Apologizing

Juliana Breines, "When 'I'm Sorry' Is Too Much," *Psychology Today*, June 24, 2013.

Sorry I don't have more sources here.

Multitasking

Travis Bradberry, "Multitasking Damages Your Brain and Career, New Stud- ies Suggest," *Forbes*, October 8, 2014.

Adam Gorlick, "Media Multitaskers Pay Mental Price, Stanford Study Shows," Stanford.edu, August 24, 2009. http://news.stanford.edu/news/2009 /august24/multitask-research-study-082409.html

G. Mark et al., *Bored Mondays and Focused Afternoons: The Rhythm of Attention and Online Activity in the Workplace*. Proceedings of the SIGCHI Confer- ence on Human Factors in Computing Systems, ACM Press, 2014.

———, *Stress and Multitasking In Everyday College Life: An Empirical Study of Online Activity*, Proceedings of the SIGCHI Conference on Human Factors in Computing Systems, ACM Press, 2014.

"The Myth of Multitasking," NPR, May 10, 2013. www.npr.org/2013/05/10 /182861382/the-myth-of-multitasking

"Ten Rules for Writing Fiction," *Guardian*, February 19, 2010.

Eye contact

"Eye Contact May Make People More Resistant to Persuasion," *Science Daily*, October 2, 2013. www.sciencedaily.com/releases/2013/10/131002092629 .htm?utm_source=feedburner&utm_medium=feed&utm_campaign =Feed%3A+sciencedaily+(ScienceDaily%3A+Latest+Science+News)

Happiness

J. Gruber, I. B. Mauss, and M. Tamir, "A Dark Side of Happiness? How, When and Why Happiness Is Not Always Good." *Perspectives on Psychological Science*, 2011.

Anna North, "Beware of Joy," *New York Times*, September 29, 2014.

Meditation

Mary Garden, "Can Meditation Be Bad for You?" *Humanist*, August 22, 2007.

Markus MacGill, "Meditation Has 'Some Benefit Against Anxiety, Depression and Pain,'" *Medical News Today*, January 7, 2014. www.medicalnewstoday .com/articles/270824.php

Self-help Books

"Can Self-Help Be Bad for You?" NHS.uk, July 6, 2009. www.nhs.uk/news/2009 /07July/Pages/SelfHelpCanBeBad.aspx

Jason Hanna, "Good, Bad and Ugly Self-Help: How Can You Tell?" CNN .com, December 7, 2009. www.cnn.com/2009/LIVING/12/07/self.help /index.html?iref=24hours

Kate Linthicum and DeeDee Correll, "Self-Help Guru Arrested in Arizona Sweat Lodge Deaths," *Los Angeles Times*, February 4, 2010.

John C. Norcross et al., *Self-Help That Works: Resources to Improve Emotional Health and Strengthen Relationships*, Oxford University Press, 2013.

Gabriele Oettingen, "The Problem with Positive Thinking," *New York Times*, October 24, 2014.

MEDICINE
Multivitamins

Paul Offit, "The Vitamin Myth: Why We Think We Need Supplements," *Atlantic*, July 19, 2013.

Nancy Shute, "The Case Against Multivitamins Grows Stronger," NPR, December 17, 2013. www.npr.org/blogs/health/2013/12/17/251955878/the-case -against-multivitamins-grows-stronger

Megan Thielking, "How a Crazy Scientist Duped America into Believing Vitamin C Cures Colds," *Vox.com*, January 15, 2015. www.vox.com/2015/1/15 /7547741/vitamin-c-myth-pauling

Annual Physicals

Jane Brody, "A Check on Physicals," *New York Times*, January 21, 2013.

Ezekiel Emanuel, "Skip Your Annual Physical," *New York Times*, January 8, 2015.

Linda Marsa, "Annual Checkups Are a Waste of Time," *Discover*, March 19, 2013.

Elisabeth Rosenthal, "Let's (Not) Get Physicals," *New York Times*, June 2, 2012.

Aspirin

"A Daily Aspirin Might Do More Harm Than Good," *Telegraph*, February 15, 2015.

"Is Taking a Daily Low-Dose Aspirin Safe for You?" *Harvard Health Publications*, October 2012.

Roni Caryn Rabin, "How Much Aspirin Is Too Much of a Good Thing?" *New York Times*, March 26, 2012.

Anna Wilde Mathews, "The Danger of Taking Aspirin Daily," *Wall Street Journal*, February 23, 2010.

Mammograms

Salynn Boyles, "New Mammogram Screening Guidelines FAQ," WebMD.com, accessed February 14, 2015. www.webmd.com/breast-cancer/features/new-mammogram-screening-guidelines-faq

Otis Brawley, "Mammograms: Are They Needed or Not?" CNN.com, February 20, 2014. www.cnn.com/2014/02/19/health/mammogram-studies/

Bahar Gholipour, "Mammograms Do Not Reduce Breast Cancer Deaths, Study Finds," *Foxnews.com*, February 12, 2014. www.foxnews.com/health/2014/02/12/mammograms-do-not-reduce-breast-cancer-deaths-study-finds/

Gina Kolata, "Vast Study Casts Doubts on Value of Mammograms," *New York Times*, February 11, 2014.

Sandhya Pruthi, "Mammogram Guidelines: What's Changed?" MayoClinic.com, Answers from May 3, 2013. www.mayoclinic.org/tests-procedures/mammogram/expert-answers/mammogram guidelines/faq 20057759

Teeth Brushing

Jennifer Berman, "Kale? Juicing? Trouble Ahead," *New York Times*, January 1, 2014.

Melissa Breyer, "Could Brushing Right After a Meal Be Bad for Your Teeth?" *Huffington Post*, November 5, 2013. www.huffingtonpost.com/2013/11/05 /brush-teeth-after-meal_n_4173794.html

Anahad O'Connor, "Really? Never Brush Your Teeth Immediately After a Meal," *New York Times*, May 21, 2012.

Statins

Gretchen Reynolds, "Can Statins Cut the Benefits of Exercise?" *New York Times*, May 22, 2013.

Peter Russell, "Why Statins Might Raise Diabetes Risk," WebMD.com, September 24, 2014. www.webmd.com/cholesterol-management/news/20140924/statins -diabetes-risk

Gianluigi Savarese et al., "Benefits of Statins in Elderly Subjects Without Established Cardiovascular Disease," *Journal of the American College of Cardiology*, December 2013, doi:10.1016/J.Jacc.2013.07.069.

Q-tips

"AAO-HNSF Clinical Practice Guideline: Earwax Removal," Entnet.org, August 29, 2008. www.entnet.org/content/aao-hnsf-clinical-practice-guideline-earwax -removal

William Brennan, "Should You Use Q-Tips to Clean Your Ears?" *Slate*, March 11, 2013.

Sarah Klein, "This Will Make You Never, Ever Want to Clean Your Ears Again," *Huffington Post*, July 21, 2014. www.huffingtonpost.com/2014/07/21/dont -clean-ear-qtip_n_5600401.html

Blood Pressure Drugs

Kathryn Doyle, "Blood Pressure Meds May Raise Elderly Fall Risk," *Reuters*, February 26, 2014.

Anahad O'Connor, "Blood Pressure Drugs Tied to Risk of Falls," *New York Times*, February 24, 2014.

"High Blood Pressure Dangers: Hypertension's Effects on the Body," MayoClinic.com, February 18, 2014.

New Medical Procedures

Nicholas Bakalar, "Medical Procedures May Be Useless, or Worse," *New York Times*, July 26, 2013.

Otis Brawley, *How We Do Harm: A Doctor Breaks Ranks About Being Sick in America*, St. Martin's Griffin, 2012.

Herbal Supplements

"Herbal Supplements: What to Know Before You Buy," MayoClinic.com, November 17, 2011. www.mayoclinic.org/healthy-lifestyle/nutrition-and-healthy-eating/in-depth/herbal-supplements/art-20046714

Geoffrey Kabat, "Natural Does Not Mean Safe," *Slate*, November 26, 2012.

Eric Lipton, "Support Is Mutual for Senator and Utah Industry," *New York Times*, June 20, 2011.

Donald Marcus, "The Consequences of Ineffective Regulation of Dietary Supplements," *Journal of American Medical Association*, July 9, 2012, doi:10.1001/Archinternmed.2012.2687.

Yvette Terrie, "Herbal Supplements May Not Be As Safe As They Sound," *U.S. News and World Report*, June 22, 2013.

DRINK
Diet Soda

Allison Aubrey, "Could Diet Soda Really Be Better Than Water for Weight Loss?" NPR.com, May 28, 2014. www.npr.org/blogs/thesalt/2014/05/28/316321004/industry-study-finds-diet-drinks-help-dieters-shed-more-lbs-than-water

Sallyn Boyles, with Laura J. Martin, "Does Diet Soda Really Cause Weight Gain? What Experts Say," WebMD.com, November 29, 2010. www.webmd.com/diet/diet-sodas-and-weight-gain-not-so-fast

Kenneth Chang, "Artificial Sweeteners May Disrupt Body's Blood Sugar Controls," *New York Times*, September 17, 2014.

Quentin Fottrell, "How Diet Soda Can Sabotage Your Diet," MarketWatch.com, June 30, 2014. www.marketwatch.com/story/how-diet-soda-can-sabotage-your-diet-2014-06-27

Water

Coco Ballantyne, "Strange But True: Drinking Too Much Water Can Kill," *Scientific American*, June 21, 2007.

Deborah Blum, "A Heart Risk in Drinking Water," *New York Times*, 2014.

Gina Kolata, "Marathoners Warned About Too Much Water," *New York Times*, October 20, 2005.

Mayo Clinic Staff, "Water: How Much Should You Drink Every Day?" MayoClinic.com, September 5, 2014. www.mayoclinic.org/healthy-lifestyle /nutrition-and-healthy-eating/in-depth/water/art-20044256

Lara Rosenbaum, "Are You Overhydrated?" MensHealth.com, September 12, 2014. www.menshealth.com/health/overhydration-dangers

Fruit Juice

Esther Crain, "Is Fruit Juice Any Healthier Than a Can of Soda?" *Women's Health*, February 10, 2014.

Jason M. R. Gill and Naveed Sattar, "Fruit Juice: Just Another Sugary Drink?" TheLancet.com, February 10, 2014, doi: http://dx.doi.org/10.1016/S2213 -8587(14)70013-0.

Milk

Aaron Carroll, "Got Milk? Might Not Be Doing You Much Good," *New York Times*, November 17, 2014.

Faye Flam, "Holy Cow! Study Suggests Milk Is Bad for Bones, Heart. Has the Medical Establishment Lied to Us?" Forbes.com, October 30, 2014. www .forbes.com/sites/fayeflam/2014/10/30/holy-cow-study-suggests-milk-is -bad-for-bones-heart-has-the-medical-establishment-lied-to-us/

David Katz, "Milk and Mortality: Questioning the Answers," *U.S. News and World Report*, November 3, 2014.

Maggie Lange, "Heroic Study Says Milk Is Bad for Women," *New York*, October 29, 2014. http://nymag.com/thecut/2014/10/heroic-study-says-milk-is-bad -for-women.html

Dennis Thompson, "Is Milk Your Friend or Foe?" WebMD.com, October 29, 2014. www.webmd.com/osteoporosis/news/20141029/is-milk-your-friend -or-foe

Green Tea

Tod Cooperman, "Warning . . . Your Green Tea Isn't What You Think It Is," *BottomLineHealth.com*, September 1, 2013. http://bottomlinehealth.com /warningyour-green-tea-isnt-what-you-think-it-is/

Susi May, "Is It Possible to Drink Too Much Green Tea?" Health.com, August 20, 2013. http://news.health.com/2013/08/20/is-it-possible-to-drink-too-much -green-tea/

Laura Newcomer, "13 Reasons Tea Is Good for You," *Time*, September 4, 2012.

Anahad O'Connor, "What's in Your Green Tea?" *New York Times*, May 23, 2013.

"Tea Addiction Results in Woman's Tooth Loss," *Huffington Post*, March 21, 2013. www.huffingtonpost.com/2013/03/21/tea-addiction-tooth-loss_n _2925013.html

Breast-Feeding Instead of Baby Formula

Nicholas Bakalar, "Is Breast-Feeding Really Better?" *New York Times*, March 4, 2014.

Emily Caldwell, "Breast-Feeding Benefits Appear to Be Overstated, According to Study of Siblings," Ohio State University, ResearchNews.osu.edu, February 25, 2014. http://researchnews.osu.edu/archive/sibbreast.htm

Cynthia Colen and D. M. Ramey, "Is Breast Truly Best? Estimating the Effects of Breast-feeding on Long-Term Child Health and Wellbeing in the United States Using Sibling Comparisons," *Social Science & Medicine*, May 2014, doi: 10.1016/j.socscimed.2014.01.027.

Mayo Clinic Staff, "Breast-Feeding Versus Formula-Feeding: What's Best?" MayoClinic.com, April 10, 2012. www.mayoclinic.org/healthy-lifestyle/infant -and-toddler-health/in-depth/breast-feeding/art-20047898

Juice Cleanse

Melinda Beck, "The Debate over Juice Cleanses and Toxin Removal," *Wall Street Journal*, March 3, 2014.

Katy Waldman, "Stop Juicing: It's Not Healthy, It's Not Virtuous, and It Makes You Seem like a Jerk," *Slate*, November 20, 2013. www.slate.com/articles /double_x/doublex/2013/11/juice_cleanses_not_healthy_not_virtuous_just _expensive.html

Vitaminwater

Susanna Kim, "Vitaminwater Lawsuit to Move Forward as Class Action," ABCnews.com, July 19, 2013. http://abcnews.go.com/Business/court-rules -vitaminwater-lawsuit-move-forward/story?id=19714482

Anahad O'Connor, "Are Vitamin Drinks a Bad Idea?" *New York Times*, January 30, 2015.

Eric Spitznagel, "Drink Deception and the Legal War on Vitaminwater," Businessweek.com, July 26, 2013. www.bloomberg.com/bw/articles/2013-07-26 /drink-deception-and-the-legal-war-on-vitaminwater

FITNESS
Stand-Up Desks

A. J. Jacobs, *Drop Dead Healthy: One Man's Humble Quest for Bodily Perfection*, Simon & Schuster, 2012.

"Women Are Piling on the Pounds Because They Have Cut Down on Housework, Study Shows," *Daily Mail*, February 28, 2013.

Ball Chairs

Gretchen Reynolds, "Ask Well: Do Ball Chairs Offer Benefits?" *New York Times*, April 12, 2013.

Stretching

Gretchen Reynolds, "Reasons Not to Stretch," *New York Times*, April 3, 2013.

Diets

Renée Atallah et al., "Long-Term Effects of 4 Popular Diets on Weight Loss and Cardiovascular Risk Factors," *Circulation: Cardiovascular Quality and Outcomes*, November 11, 2014, doi: 10.1161/Circoutcomes.113.000723.

Daniel J. DeNoon, "Diets Don't Work Long-Term," WebMD.com, April 11, 2007. www.webmd.com/diet/20070411/diets-dont-work-long-term

"Study: Popular Diets Don't Work in the Long-Term," *Today Show*, November 12, 2014.

Infomercial Fitness Products

Nicholas Bakalar, "The Unproven Claims of Fitness Products," *New York Times*, July 23, 2012.

Carl Heneghan et al., "The Evidence Underpinning Sports Performance Products: A Systematic Assessment," *BMJ Open*, 2012;2:e001702, doi:10.1136/bmjopen-2012-001702.

Yoga

William Broad, the *Science of Yoga: The Risks and the Rewards*, Simon & Schuster, 2012.

Paige Greenfield, "Will Yoga Really Wreck Your Body?" *Men's Health*, January 20, 2012.

Cross-fit

Christie Aschwanden, "An Insider's Guide to Cross-fit, *New York Times*, August 18, 2014.

Ken Reed, "Cross-fit: Too Much of a Good Thing Is Definitely Bad," *Huffington Post*, March 30, 2014. www.huffingtonpost.com/ken-reed/crossfit_b_4666040.html

Mark Rippetoe, "Cross-fit: The Good, the Bad and the Ugly," *Huffington Post*, December 10, 2013. www.huffingtonpost.com/mark-rippetoe/crossfit-good-bad-ugly_b_4420922.html

Mark Rippetoe, *Starting Strength*, 3rd ed., Aasgaard Company, 2011.

Exercise

Jessica Firger, "Too Much Exercise May Be Bad for the Heart," CBSnews.com, May 14, 2014. www.cbsnews.com/news/too-much-exercise-may-be-bad-for-the-heart/

Heart and Vascular Team, "Can Too Much Extreme Exercise Damage Your Heart?" Health.Cleveland.Clinic.org, September 11, 2014. http://health.clevelandclinic.org/2014/09/can-too-much-extreme-exercise-damage-your-heart/

Kevin Helliker, "The Exercise Equivalent of a Cheeseburger?" *Wall Street Journal*, May 14, 2013.

———, "Too Much Exercise May Be Harmful to Your Health," *Wall Street Journal*, May 14, 2014.

Gretchen Reynolds, "Can You Get Too Much Exercise?" *New York Times*, July 24, 2013.

———, "Exercising But Gaining Weight," *New York Times*, November 12, 2014.

———, "Is Exercise Bad for Your Teeth?" *New York Times*, September 24, 2014.

———, "Is Marathon Running Bad for the Heart?" *New York Times*, May 23, 2012.

Alexandra Sifferlin, "Is Exercise Harmful for Some People?" *Time*, June 1, 2012.

EVERYTHING ELSE

Marriage

Phil Hammond, "Are Relationships Good or Bad for Your Health?" *Telegraph*, June 2, 2014.

Jonathan Gardner and Andrew Oswald, "How Is Mortality Affected By Money, Marriage and Stress?" *Journal of Health Economics* 23 (2004): 1181–1207.

Claire Miller, "Study Finds More Reasons to Get and Stay Married," *New York Times*, January 8, 2015.

Tara Parker-Pope, "The Happy Marriage Is the 'Me' Marriage," *New York Times*, December 31, 2010.

Theresa Tamkins, "Unhappily Ever After: Why Bad Marriages Hurt Women's Health," CNN.com, March 6, 2009. www.cnn.com/2009/HEALTH/03/06/marriage.women.heart/index.html?iref=24hours

Choice

Walter Isaacson, *Steve Jobs*, Simon & Schuster, 2012.

Sheena Iyengar, Rachael Wells, and Barry Schwartz, "Doing Better But Feeling Worse," *Association for Psychological Science* 17, no. 2 (2006): 143–150.

Ian Kerner, "Dating and the Challenge of Too Many Choices," CNN.com, January 26, 2012. http://thechart.blogs.cnn.com/2012/01/26/dating-and-the-challenge-of-too-many-choices/

Barry Schwartz, *The Paradox of Choice: Why More Is Less*, Harper Perennial, 2005.

News

Rolf Dobelli, "News Is Bad for You—and Giving Up Reading It Will Make You Happier," *Guardian*, April 12, 2013.

Jon Hamilton, "Bingeing on Bad News Can Fuel Daily Stress," NPR, July 10, 2014. www.npr.org/blogs/health/2014/07/10/323355132/binging-on-bad-news-can-fuel-daily-stress

Melissa Healy, "Toll of Disturbing News Is Greater for Women, Study Says," *Los Angeles Times*, October 12, 2012.

E. Alison Holman, Dana Rose Garfin, and Roxane Cohen Silver, "Media's Role in Broadcasting Acute Stress Following the Boston Marathon Bombings," *Proceedings of the National Academy of Sciences* 111, no. 1 (2013): 93–98, doi: 10.1073/pnas.1316265110.

Marie-France Marin et al., "There Is No News Like Bad News: Women Are More Remembering and Stress Reactive After Reading Real Negative News Than Men," *PLOS One*, October 10, 2012, doi: 10.1371/journal.pone.0047189.

College Degrees

Brooke Berger, "Why a College Degree May Not Be Worth It," *U.S. News and World Report*, May 9, 2013.

"Is College Worth It?" *Economist*, April 5, 2014.

Jacques Steinberg, "Plan B: Skip College," *New York Times*, May 15, 2010.

Height

Brian Palmer, "The Research Is Clear: Being Tall Is Hazardous to Your Health," *Slate*, July 30, 2013.

Tara Parker-Pope, "Cancer Risk Increases with Height," *New York Times*, July 25, 2013.

Alexandra Sifferlin, "How Height Is Connected to Cancer," *Time*, July 26, 2013.

Retirement

American Institute of Stress, "Holmes-Rahe Stress Inventory," www.stress.org/holmes-rahe-stress-inventory/, accessed June 10, 2014.

Moderation

Stephen H. Boutcher, "High-Intensity Intermittent Exercise and Fat Loss," *Journal of Obesity*, November 24, 2010, doi: 10.1155/2011/868305.

Jeremy Duvall, "8 Amazing Fat Burning Intervals," MensFitness.com, accessed February 7, 2015. www.mensfitness.com/training/cardio/8-amazing-fat -burning-intervals

Alexandra Sifferlin, "Short Bursts of Exercise Are Better Than Exercising Nonstop," *Time*, August 5, 2014.

Laughter

R. E. Ferner and J. K. Aronson, "Laughter and Mirth (Methodical Investigation of Risibility, Therapeutic and Harmful): Narrative Synthesis," *BMJ* 2013;347, doi: http://dx.doi.org/10.1136/bmj.F7274.

Jan Hoffman, "Who Says Laughter's the Best Medicine?" *New York Times*, December 20, 2013.

FINAL THOUGHTS

Abby Ellin, "What's Eating Our Kids? Fears About 'Bad' Foods," *New York Times*, February 25, 2009.

Sumathi Reddy, "When Healthy Eating Calls for Treatment," *Wall Street Journal*, November 10, 2014.

Acknowledgments

The true visionary behind this book is Bob Miller, Flatiron's publisher and fearless leader, who noticed that every week, there seemed to be a new study saying *"Bad Thing* is now good!" or *"Good Thing* is now bad!" The book started with him. Thank you, Bob, for trusting me with your idea, and for shepherding it from concept to reality.

I never would have been connected to Bob without my incredible agent, Rob Weisbach. Thank you, Rob, for providing unflagging support, perspective, advice, and for being one of the most authentic and nicest people I've ever met. Many thanks to editor Jasmine Faustino for her sharp eye, consistently great insights, and amazing ability to somehow inpose order on my chaos. Thanks for keeping me honest, Jasmine. Thanks to attorney Henry Kaufman for the legal read to keep me out of jail (good news about something else that's bad for you: lawyers). Thanks to the phenomenal team at Flatiron, including associate publisher Liz Keenan, publicity

superstar Steven Boriack, marketing manager Molly Fonseca, managing editor David Lott, production editor John Morrone, production manager Eric Gladstone, the amazing (and patient!) designer Michelle McMillian, and Karen Horton, the brains behind the book's dueling covers. (And thanks to whoever mailed me that Flatiron coffee mug. I use it.)

This book, naturally, leans heavily on the health experts that I interviewed. You're all rock stars. (But smarter and better educated.) At the risk of droning on like an Oscars awards speech or, worse, forgetting someone, thank you to Alan Hedge, Allan Brett, Andrew Newberg, Barry Schwartz, Brett Ford, Carol Goman, David Allison, David Katz, David Tovey, Denise Pope, Donald Marcus, Duane Knudson, Gloria Mark, Gretchen Reynolds, John Norcross, Joseph Verbalis, Karina Schumann, Katherine Beals, Liz Applegate, Mark Haub, Nancy Rojas, Nina Teicholz, Robert Delamontagne, Robert London, Steven Salzberg, Stuart Lewis, Susan Swithers, Ivan Oransky, Thomas Dunn, and the countless scientists, doctors, researchers, and writers of health articles that informed this book.

Thanks to those who read early drafts and helped sharpen and improve them, including my old coauthor Andrea Syrtash, Jen Doll, Braxton Robbason, Lindsay Crouse, Laura Brounstein, Trevor Hoff, Tania Hoff, Laura Demoreuille, Rochelle Bilow, Carolyn Murnick, Carmella Tress, and Wes Hollomon.

As every writer knows, you get a lot of your ideas by talking to friends and family and coworkers. This book is no different. Especially since the scope is so broad, I've been lucky enough to get a *lot* of inspiration from smart people who I'm lucky to have in my life. My parents and stepparents, sisters and brother, aunts, uncles, and cousins: thank you. All of you. Special thanks to Keith Meatto, Leo Lopez, Lee Bob Black, Joe Hall, Eric Pedersen, Cody Dolan, Dan

Abbruscato, Jamie Davis, Evan Aronowitz, Walker Robinson, James Mangano, Charlie Applegate, Stephen Murray, Terry Selucky, Amy Braunschweiger, Annie Shapero, Adam Smith, Stephane Conte, Dave Spinks, Erik Brown, Lindsay #yolo, Matt Smith, Teddy Vuong, Meredith T, Curtis Sparrer, Kabir Merchant, Todd Rinaldo, Stephanie Meyers, Paul Jarrett, Alyssa Shelasky, Laura Strausfeld, Brad Cohen, Jo, Michael Sang, Betsy Poris, Juliet Nuss, Harry McNeil, Traci Swain, Ann-Marie Resnick, Ellie Chamberland, Wayne Friedman, and the rest of the mighty crew at Scholastic. Thanks to the old faithful Wednesday night Writer's Group, including Shawn Regruto, Lisa Ebersole, Maya Singer, Jared Roberts, Damien Paris, Lisa Schiller, Andrea Miller, and the rest of you brilliant and beautiful people at The Table.

And thank you to everyone—including you, the reader—for putting up with what I'll call the "Cliff Clavin" problem. Remember *Cheers*? Cliff loved to share dumb little factoids. It was insufferable. "Hey, Normie, you know, the Portuguese once conducted a study, finding that the health benefits of potatoes—" After spending months and months researching this book, I've developed something of a Cliff Clavin Problem. I can't stop sharing dumb little factoids about health. So, thanks for indulging me.

And then, finally, thank you to all the makers of whiskey, beer, and bacon. Clearly you're making the world a healthier place.

Index